Glaucoma

ESASO Course Series

Vol. 8

Series Editors

F. Bandello Milan
B. Corcóstegui Barcelona

Glaucoma

Volume Editors

Carlo E. Traverso Genoa
Ingeborg Stalmans Leuven
Fotis Topouzis Thessaloniki
Luca Bagnasco Genoa

64 figures, 46 in color, and 17 tables, 2016

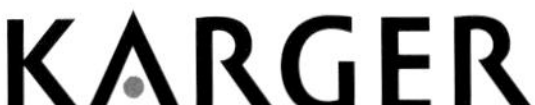

Basel · Freiburg · Paris · London · New York · Chennai · New Delhi ·
Bangkok · Beijing · Shanghai · Tokyo · Kuala Lumpur · Singapore · Sydney

Carlo E. Traverso
Clinica Oculistica, Di.N.O.G.M.I. University of Genoa
and IRCCS Azienda Ospedaliera Universitaria
San Martino IST
Viale Benedetto XV 7
IT–16132 Genoa (Italy)

Ingeborg Stalmans
Department of Ophthalmology
Glaucoma Clinic
University Hospitals Leuven UZ Leuven
Herestraat 49
BE–3000 Leuven (Belgium)

Fotis Topouzis
Laboratory of Research and Clinical
Applications in Ophthalmology
A' Department of Ophthalmology
Aristotle University of Thessaloniki
AHEPA Hospital
Stilponos Kyriakidi 1
GR–54636 Thessaloniki (Greece)

Luca Bagnasco
Clinica Oculistica, Di.N.O.G.M.I.
University of Genoa
Viale Benedetto XV 7
IT–16132 Genoa (Italy)

Library of Congress Cataloging-in-Publication Data

Names: Traverso, Carlo E., editor. | Stalmans, Ingeborg, editor. | Topouzis,
    Fotis, editor. | Bagnasco, Luca, editor. | European School for Advanced
    Studies in Ophthalmology, issuing body.
Title: Glaucoma / volume editors, Carlo E. Traverso, Ingeborg Stalmans, Fotis
    Topouzis, Luca Bagnasco.
Other titles: Glaucoma (Traverso) | ESASO course series ; v. 8. 1664-882X
Description: Basel ; New York : Karger, 2016. | Series: ESASO course series,
    ISSN 1664-882X ; vol. 8 | Includes bibliographical references and index.
Identifiers: LCCN 2016034669| ISBN 9783318058901 (hard cover : alk. paper) |
    ISBN 9783318058918 (e-ISBN)
Subjects: | MESH: Glaucoma
Classification: LCC RE871 | NLM WW 290 | DDC 617.7/41--dc23 LC record available at https://lccn.loc.gov/2016034669

Contents

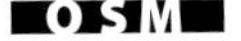

Online supplementary material: www.karger.com/book/toc/271780

Preface

The Glaucoma Module of the ESASO can be defined as a group of interactive lectures spanning extensively into the various topics of glaucoma diagnosis and care. This book contains the written form of the Module, with the advantage of being always accessible and the disadvantage of not allowing direct interaction with the experts. The practical clinical approach, however, is suitably transferred from the lectures, leaving the reader with additional bits of knowledge that can be used to manage real patients during their real professional activity.

All authors are to be commended for committing to this exercise, which was demanding both in time and in energy. I believe that the ambitious goal of being concise and focused has been achieved here, thanks also to the scientific coordinators Fotis Topouzis and Ingeborg Stalmans.

I trust this book will provide fruitful reading and an up-to-date review on glaucoma. The commitment and support of the ESASO Board for this project is also gratefully acknowledged.

Carlo Enrico Traverso, Genoa

List of Contributors

Alessandro Bagnis
Clinica Oculistica, Di.N.O.G.M.I.
University of Genoa and
IRCCS Azienda Ospedaliera
Universitaria San Martino IST
Viale Benedetto XV 7
IT–16132 Genoa (Italy)
E-Mail alebagnis@libero.it

Rupert R.A. Bourne
Vision and Eye Research Unit
Anglia Ruskin University
East Road
Cambridge CB1 1PT (UK)
E-Mail rb@rupertbourne.co.uk

Paolo Brusini
Glaucoma Unit
Città di Udine Health Center
Viale Venezia 410
IT–33100 Udine (Italy)
E-Mail brusini@libero.it

Carlo Alberto Cutolo
Clinica Oculistica, Di.N.O.G.M.I.
University of Genoa and
IRCCS Azienda Ospedaliera
Universitaria San Martino IST
Viale Benedetto XV 7
IT–16132 Genoa (Italy)
E-Mail cacutolo@gmail.com

Barbara Cvenkel
Department of Ophthalmology
University Medical Center Ljubljana
Grablovičeva 46
SI–1000 Ljubljana (Slovenia)
E-Mail barbara.cvenkel@gmail.com

Panayiota Founti
Moorfields Eye Hospital
Flat 1, 105 Holloway Road
London N7 8LT (UK)
E-Mail pfounti@gmail.com

Pelagia Kalouda
Laboratory of Research and Clinical
Applications in Ophthalmology
A' Department of Ophthalmology
Aristotle University of Thessaloniki
AHEPA Hospital
Stilponos Kyriakidi 1
GR–54636 Thessaloniki (Greece)
E-Mail pelkalouda@gmail.com

Christina Keskini
Laboratory of Research and Clinical
Applications in Ophthalmology
A' Department of Ophthalmology
Aristotle University of Thessaloniki
AHEPA Hospital
Stilponos Kyriakidi 1
GR–54636 Thessaloniki (Greece)
E-Mail chr.1987@hotmail.com

Aachal Kotecha
Visual Neuroscience Laboratory
UCL Institute of Ophthalmology
11–43 Bath Street
London EC1V 9EL (UK)
E-Mail aachalkotecha@moorfields.nhs.uk

Alexander Spratt
Beraja Medical Institute
2550 South Douglas Road
Miami, FL 33131 (USA)
E-Mail alexspratt@gmail.com

Ingeborg Stalmans
Department of Ophthalmology
Glaucoma Clinic
University Hospitals Leuven UZ Leuven
Herestraat 49
BE–3000 Leuven (Belgium)
E-Mail ingeborg.stalmans@uzleuven.be

John Thygesen
Department of Ophthalmology
Rigshospitalet
Copenhagen University Hospital
Nordre Ringvej 57
DK–2600 Glostrup (Denmark)
E-Mail john.thygesen@regionh.dk

Fotis Topouzis
Laboratory of Research and Clinical
Applications in Ophthalmology
A' Department of Ophthalmology
Aristotle University of Thessaloniki
AHEPA Hospital
Stilponos Kyriakidi 1
GR–54636 Thessaloniki (Greece)
E-Mail ftopou12@otenet.gr

Carlo Enrico Traverso
Clinica Oculistica, Di.N.O.G.M.I.
University of Genoa and
IRCCS Azienda Ospedaliera
Universitaria San Martino IST
Viale Benedetto XV 7
IT–16132 Genoa (Italy)
E-Mail mc8620@mclink.it

Ananth Viswanathan
Glaucoma Service
Moorfields Eye Hospital
32 Eagle Wharf
138 Grosvenor Road
London SW1V 3JS (UK)
E-Mail a.viswanathan@ucl.ac.uk

Traverso CE, Stalmans I, Topouzis F, Bagnasco L (eds): Glaucoma.
ESASO Course Series. Basel, Karger, 2016, vol 8, pp 1–8 (DOI: 10.1159/000446132)

Imaging for Glaucoma Detection and Progression

Rupert R.A. Bourne

Vision and Eye Research Unit, Anglia Ruskin University, and Addenbrooke's Hospital, Cambridge, and Hinchingbrooke Hospital, Huntingdon, UK

Abstract

All types of glaucoma involve glaucomatous optic neuropathy. The key to the detection and management of glaucoma is understanding how to examine the optic nerve head (ONH). The rate of structural progression is highly variable with some individuals progressing very slowly over many years, while others exhibit a much more rapidly progressing picture. This talk covers a series of related topics, the characteristics of a normal and a glaucomatous ONH, the strategies by which to measure progression (clinical judgement, event, and trend analysis), and instruments that can assist the clinician in the detection and monitoring of structural progression (ONH photography, optical coherence tomography, and confocal scanning laser ophthalmoscopy). The talk is illustrated with examples of clinical imaging, and suggestions for further reading are given. © 2016 S. Karger AG, Basel

Introduction

All types of glaucoma involve glaucomatous optic neuropathy. The key to detection and management of glaucoma is understanding how to examine the optic nerve head (ONH) [1]. The rate of structural progression is highly variable with some individuals progressing very slowly over many years, while others exhibit a much more rapidly progressing picture.

This talk covers a series of related topics: normal characteristics of the ONH, characteristics of a glaucomatous ONH, strategies to measure progression, and instruments used for measuring structural progression.

Normal Characteristics of the Optic Nerve Head

The ONH or optic disc is a round/oval 'plughole', down which more than a million nerve fibres descend through a sieve-like sheet known as the lamina cribrosa (fig. 1). These fibres are then bundled together behind the eye as the optic nerve, which continues towards the brain. The retinal nerve fibres are spread unevenly across the surface of the retina in a thin layer, which has a 'feathery' appearance, best seen immediately above and below the disc. As the nerve fibres converge on the edge of the disc, they pour over the scleral ring (which marks the edge of the disc) and

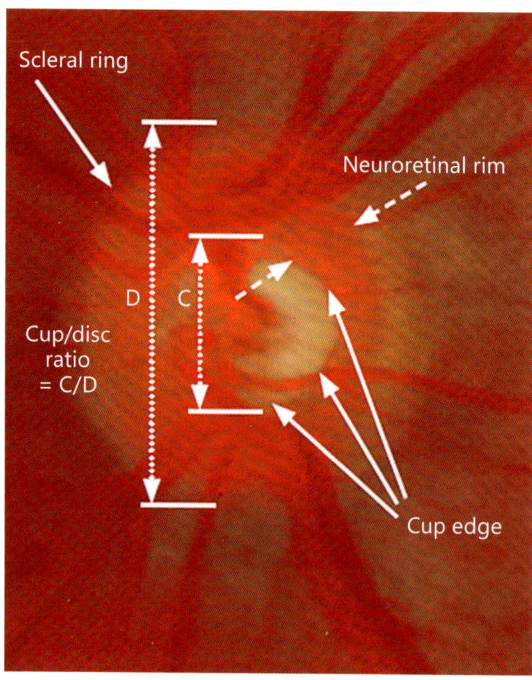

Fig. 1. Characteristics of the normal ONH.

then down its inner surface. This dense packing of nerve fibres just inside the scleral ring is visualised as the neuroretinal rim. The cup is the area central to the neuroretinal rim. The cup edge (where it meets the neuroretinal rim) is best seen by the bend in small- and medium-sized blood vessels as they descend into the cup. A colour difference should not be used to distinguish the cup edge; a change in the direction of blood vessels is a more reliable indicator. The inferior rim is usually thicker than the superior rim, which is thicker than the nasal rim, and the temporal rim is the thinnest (this is known as the ISNT rule).

Characteristics of a Glaucomatous Optic Nerve Head

Clinically observable characteristics of a glaucomatous ONH include [2]:

1 generalised/focal enlargement of the cup (fig. 2a);
2 disc haemorrhage (within 1 disc diameter of ONH) (fig. 2b);
3 thinning of the neuroretinal rim (usually at superior and inferior poles) (fig. 2c);
4 asymmetry of cupping between a patient's eyes;
5 loss of the retinal nerve fibre layer (RNFL) (fig. 2c), and
6 parapapillary atrophy (more common in glaucomatous eyes).

Various instruments are commercially available to assist in the detection of glaucomatous optic neuropathy. These include optical coherence tomography (OCT), scanning laser polarimetry, and confocal scanning laser ophthalmoscopy. The instruments give an indication of normality/abnormality of various ONH and RNFL parameters by comparing acquired measurements with those of a normative database that varies by manufacturer (fig. 3).

Strategies to Measure Progression

The appearance of any of the features of a glaucomatous ONH, or the exacerbation of these features compared to a previous record, is indicative of progression or worsening of the disease.

The speed or manner of structural progression is poorly understood with opinion divided on whether progression occurs as a continuous linear process where tissue and function are gradually affected, or as a stepwise process where an acute event causes sudden structural damage that is followed by a period with minimal change until another acute event occurs. It is possible that both patterns may coexist in certain subpopulations or might occur in the same patient in different phases of the disease. For this reason, there are different methods to assess glaucomatous progression.

In order to determine if progression is occurring, there are three main strategies: clinical judgement, event analysis, and trend analysis.

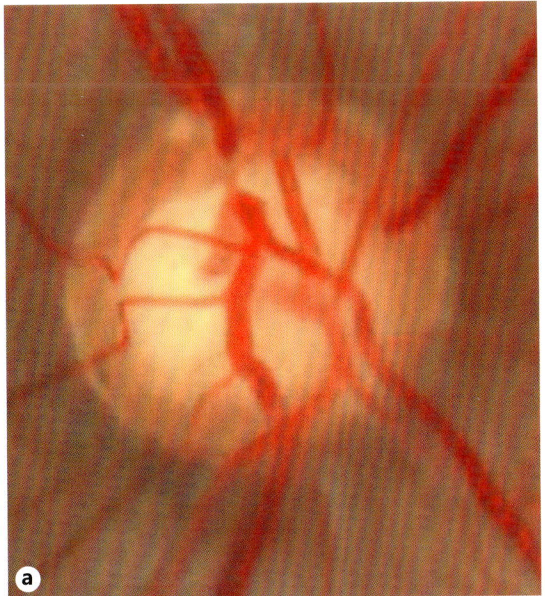
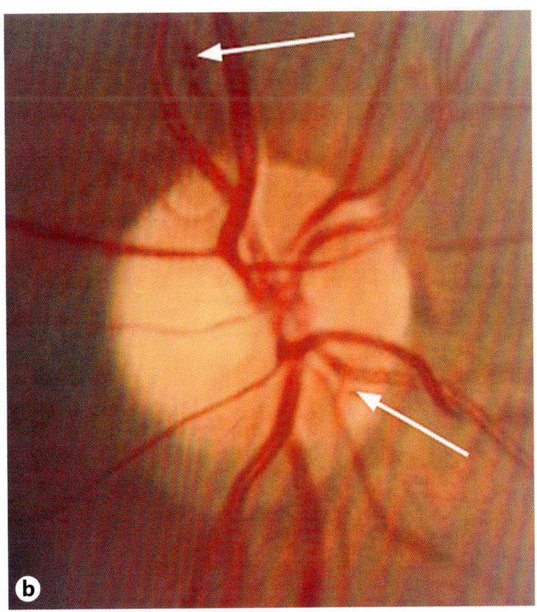
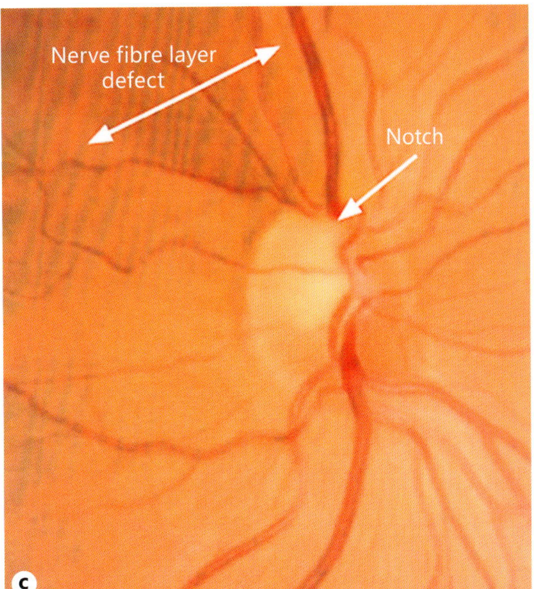

Fig. 2. Characteristics of a glaucomatous ONH. **a** Generalised enlargement of the cup. **b** Splinter haemorrhages. **c** Focal enlargement of the cup (notch) and nerve fibre layer defect.

Clinical Judgement
Clinical findings are observed over time. They are assessed subjectively. Experience of normal and glaucomatous ONH features allows one to determine if 'conversion' has occurred from a state of normality or if progression of the disease has oc-curred in an eye which already exhibits structural features of glaucoma.

Event Analysis
Progression is defined when a follow-up measurement exceeds a pre-established criterion for

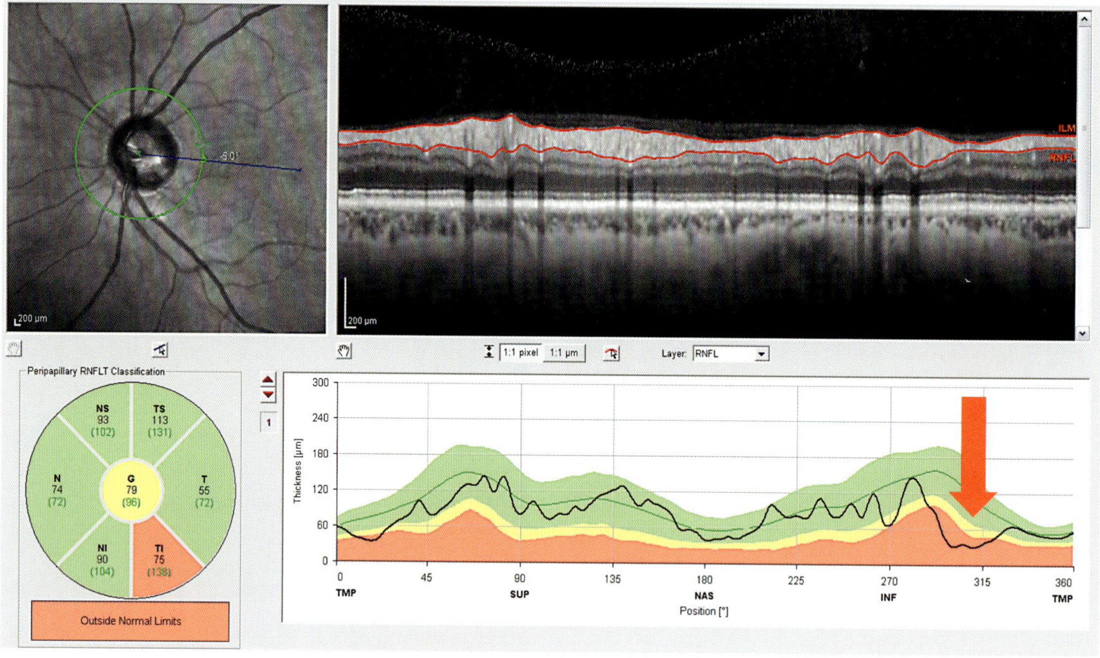

Fig. 3. ONH imaging with the SD-OCT, Heidelberg Spectralis instrument. Note the abnormally thin RNFL inferotemporal sector (marked in red).

change from baseline. It is assumed that any change below this threshold is due to natural age-related loss and/or measurement variability, while changes exceeding the threshold represent true progression. Defining the threshold for a change is an important aspect of event analysis. A higher threshold results in greater specificity because only situations with marked change will be flagged. However, this reduces sensitivity for detecting less dramatic changes. Conversely, a lower threshold improves sensitivity while simultaneously decreasing specificity. Event analysis is geared toward detecting a gradual change over time that reaches a threshold or identifying an acute event that exceeds a threshold. Event analysis is used with some imaging techniques; for example, the Heidelberg retina tomograph (HRT; Heidelberg Engineering, Heidelberg, Germany) system incorporates topographic change analysis (TCA) software (fig. 4).

Trend Analysis

Trend analysis identifies progression by monitoring the behaviour of a parameter over time. A regression analysis of a dependent variable (i.e. RNFL thickness) is performed on follow-up measurements, providing a rate of progression over time. This method is less sensitive to sudden changes and the variability among consecutive tests, as it is neutralized by the overall rate of change. Another important advantage of this method is the ability to extrapolate the rate of progression, which allows for the prediction of the time required to reach certain milestones. Trend analyses are employed by the majority of OCT instruments.

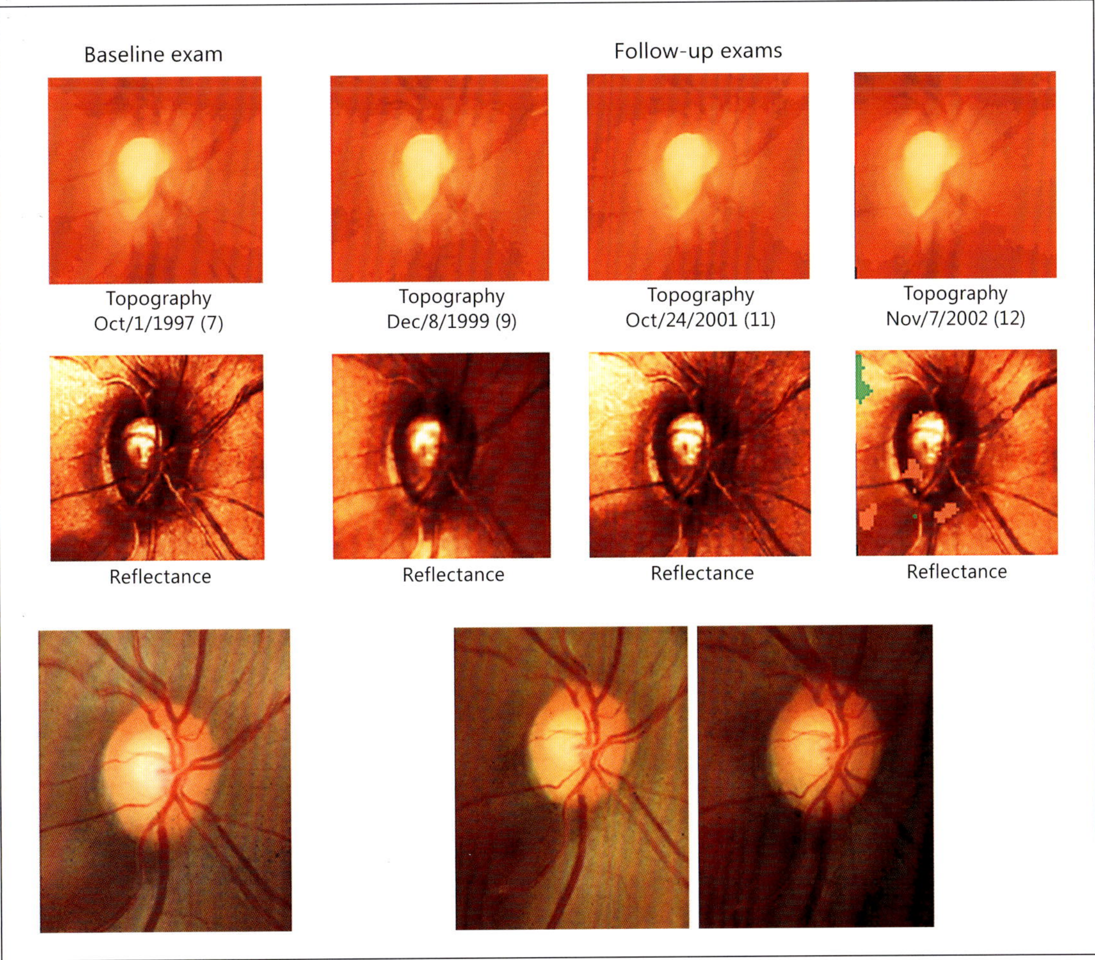

Fig. 4. HRT system TCA software. This illustration demonstrates progressive thinning of the neuroretinal rim denoted by red super-pixels. Additionally, the optic nerve photographs are shown that demonstrate concordance with the TCA findings.

Instruments Used for Measuring Structural Progression

Optic Nerve Head and Red-Free Retinal Nerve Fibre Layer Photography

Digital photography remains a valuable and enduring record of ONH features providing a contemporaneous record that is not subject to the interobserver variability seen in subjective estimates of the cup/disc ratio or hand-drawn illustrations of the disc. Stereophotography, in particular simultaneous stereo images, provide the stereoscopic clues that are so useful in judging change. Additionally, disc photography remains the only imaging technique that records the true colouring seen on clinical biomicroscopy, which is of particular importance when considering optic disc haemorrhages (which may be present for 2 weeks to 3 months and are an important prognostic sign of progression) and parapapillary atrophy (changes in β-zone parapapillary atrophy can signal glaucoma progression). These may only be visible on photographic images but not on OCT. Assessment for progressive change can be subjective for optic disc and RNFL photography [3, 4].

Optical Coherence Tomography
OCT is a high-resolution, non-contact, and non-invasive imaging technique using low-coherence interferometry to measure RNFL thickness. Spectral domain (SD)-OCT is a newer generation of OCT that offers a higher scanning rate and improved resolution (axial resolution 5–6 μm, transverse resolution 20 μm) than time domain (TD)-OCT. Due to these improvements, novel scanning patterns have been developed that deliver 3-dimensional data from areas of interest. This allows post-processing of the data in desired locations and enables registration of consecutive images. SD-OCT reduces some limitations of TD-OCT, such as the low scanning rate that makes the scans more prone to eye movement artefacts. Also, the lack of image registration with TD-OCT can result in scan misalignment and significant variability in RNFL thickness measurements, limiting one's ability to detect true structural changes over time. Strengths of OCT technology include the ability to measure structural parameters without the need for a reference plane or magnification correction, and the ability to image RNFL, ONH, and the macula.

Scanning Laser Polarimetry
Scanning laser polarimetry quantifies the peripapillary RNFL thickness along a band surrounding the ONH by analysing the birefringence properties of the retina. This device is being withdrawn commercially as OCT devices become more commonplace, although many departments still utilise this instrument principally as a diagnostic aid in situations where the RNFL is not readily visible on clinical biomicroscopy and glaucoma is suspected.

Confocal Scanning Laser Ophthalmoscopy
Confocal scanning laser ophthalmoscopy (e.g. HRT) acquires a stack of 2-dimensional scans from parallel planes. The scans are aligned to form a 3-dimensional reconstruction of the ONH and provide quantitative data of that region. The image has an axial resolution of 300 μm and transverse resolution of 10 μm.

Previous studies have shown this device to demonstrate good discriminatory ability between healthy and glaucomatous eyes.

Two progression algorithms are included in the current version of the software: trend analysis and TCA. The trend analysis can be performed for various stereometric parameters and displays normalized changes from baseline over time.

Normalisation of each parameter to a scale between –1 and +1 is done by dividing the difference between the follow-up and the baseline value by the difference between the average value for a healthy eye and an eye with advanced glaucoma. However, a formal statistical analysis of the rate of change is not provided.

TCA is an event analysis that compares the variability between baseline examinations to variability between the baseline and each follow-up examination. Changes in the topographic height of super-pixels are marked as progression if a cluster of at least 20 significantly depressed super-pixels is identified within the disc margin on 3 consecutive examinations. A height change map is generated, with areas of significant decrease in height marked in red and areas of significant increase in height marked in green (fig. 4). The depth of change corresponds with the colour saturation. The area and volume of the significantly changed regions are plotted as a function of time. Studies show that TCA can detect change by standard techniques, although the agreement is far from perfect [5–8]. HRT-TCA is the most well-developed and -tested progression analysis available for optical imaging techniques. A limitation of the TCA is the lack of clinically usable cut-offs to define progression and the inability to interpret areas of improvement (local increases in retinal height that may be associated with adjacent decreases in height).

Conclusion

A thorough understanding of the clinically observed characteristics of the normal and the glaucomatous ONH is key to determining the presence and deterioration of glaucoma. Backward compatibility is a particular issue with ONH imaging instruments when considering the use of images in a longitudinal series. This has been a particular issue with OCT imaging where RNFL thicknesses from consecutive images using different or more modern devices cannot be readily compared [9]. This limitation further highlights the importance of obtaining ONH photographs at baseline and regular intervals of follow-up.

Image quality can influence our ability to detect structural changes [10, 11]. It is therefore important to review the quality of images included in glaucomatous progression assessment. Additionally, as with visual field analysis, more than one good quality baseline image will facilitate progression analysis. Finally, several reports have noted that several structural components of longitudinal change detection that likely contribute to the variability in measurements have not been formally assessed, such as variation in clinical disc margin variability and disagreement as to what the clinician sees as the disc margin by clinical examination within clinical disc photographs and within SD-OCT B-scans [12–14]. Intersession variation and accuracy of segmentation algorithms and reference plane anatomy are beginning to be studied, but their effect on progression detection has not been formally assessed. The optimal frequency of imaging tests in following progression is unknown; however, this should be determined by considering the clinical profiles of individual patients. For example, those with advanced glaucoma may require more frequent testing as treatment reinforcement may be needed to prevent irreversible vision loss if progression is identified and confirmed. Similarly, patients who show a rapid rate of change would need more frequent monitoring to evaluate treatment response.

Suggested Reading

Glaucoma Progression: Structure and Function. Focal Points. San Francisco, American Academy of Ophthalmology, 2013.

Weinreb RN, Garway-Heath DF, Leung C, Crowston JG, Medeiros FA (eds): Progression of Glaucoma. World Glaucoma Association. Consensus Series – 8. Amsterdam, Kugler, 2011.

Welcome to the Glaucomatous Optic Neuropathy Evaluation Project! www.gone-project.com.

References

1 Bourne RR: The optic nerve head in glaucoma. Community Eye Health 2006; 19:12–13.

2 Fingeret M, Medeiros FA, Susanna R Jr, Weinreb RN: Five rules to evaluate the optic disc and retinal nerve fibre layer for glaucoma. Optometry 2005;76:661–668.

3 Hoffmann EM, Bowd C, Medeiros FA, Boden C, Grus FH, Bourne RR, Zangwill LM, Weinreb RN: Agreement among 3 optical imaging methods for the assessment of optic disc topography. Ophthalmology 2005;112:2149–2156.

4 Garway-Heath DF, Poinoosawmy D, Wollstein G, Viswanathan A, Kamal D, Fontana L, Hitchings RA: Inter- and intraobserver variation in the analysis of optic disc images: comparison of the Heidelberg retina tomograph and computer assisted planimetry. Br J Ophthalmol 1999;83:664–669.

5 Chauhan BC, Hutchison DM, Artes PH, Caprioli J, Jonas JB, LeBlanc RP, Nicolela MT: Optic disc progression in glaucoma: comparison of confocal scanning laser tomography to optic disc photographs in a prospective study. Invest Ophthalmol Vis Sci 2009;50:1682–1691.

6 Chauhan BC, McCormick TA, Nicolela MT, LeBlanc RP: Optic disc and visual field changes in a prospective longitudinal study of patients with glaucoma: comparison of scanning laser tomography with conventional perimetry and optic disc photography. Arch Ophthalmol 2001;119:1492–1499.

7 Bowd C, Balasubramanian M, Weinreb RN, Vizzeri G, Alencar LM, O'Leary N, Sample PA, Zangwill LM: Performance of confocal scanning laser tomograph topographic change analysis (TCA) for assessing glaucomatous progression. Invest Ophthalmol Vis Sci 2009;50:691–701.

8 O'Leary N, Crabb DP, Mansberger SL, Fortune B, Twa MD, Lloyd MJ, Kotecha A, Garway-Heath DF, Cioffi GA, Johnson CA: Glaucomatous progression in series of stereoscopic photographs and Heidelberg retina tomograph images. Arch Ophthalmol 2010;128:560–568.

9 Bourne RRA, Medeiros FA, Bowd C, Jahanbakhsh K, Zangwill LM, Weinreb RN: Comparability of retinal nerve fiber layer thickness measurements with optical coherence tomography instruments. Invest Ophthalmol Vis Sci 2005;46:1280–1285.

10 Zangwill L, Irak I, Berry CC, Garden V, de Souza Lima M, Weinreb RN: Effect of cataract and pupil size on image quality with confocal scanning laser ophthalmoscopy. Arch Ophthalmol 1997;115:983–990.

11 Samarawickrama C, Pai A, Huynh SC, Burlutsky G, Wong TY, Mitchell P: Influence of OCT signal strength on macular, optic nerve head, and retinal nerve fiber layer parameters. Invest Ophthalmol Vis Sci 2010;51:4471–4475.

12 Manassakorn A, Ishikawa H, Kim JS, Wollstein G, Bilonick RA, Kagemann L, Gabriele ML, Sung KR, Mumcuoglu T, Duker JS, Fujimoto JG, Schuman JS: Comparison of optic disc margin identified by color disc photography and high-speed ultrahigh-resolution optical coherence tomography. Arch Ophthalmol 2008;126:58–64.

13 Barkana Y, Harizman N, Gerber Y, Liebmann JM, Ritch R: Measurements of optic disk size with HRT II, Stratus OCT, and funduscopy are not interchangeable. Am J Ophthalmol 2006;142:375–380.

14 Strouthidis NG, Yang H, Reynaud JF, Grimm JL, Gardiner SK, Fortune B, Burgoyne CF: Comparison of clinical and spectral domain optical coherence tomography optic disc margin anatomy. Invest Ophthalmol Vis Sci 2009;50:4709–4718.

Prof. Rupert R.A. Bourne
Vision and Eye Research Unit
Anglia Ruskin University, East Road
Cambridge CB1 1PT (UK)
E-Mail rb@rupertbourne.co.uk

Traverso CE, Stalmans I, Topouzis F, Bagnasco L (eds): Glaucoma.
ESASO Course Series. Basel, Karger, 2016, vol 8, pp 9–24 (DOI: 10.1159/000446135)

Visual Field Examination in Glaucoma: Detection and Progression of Disease

Paolo Brusini

Glaucoma Unit, Città di Udine Health Center, Udine, Italy

Abstract

The visual field (VF) test is currently the most useful technique both for an unambiguous diagnosis and for the follow-up of chronic glaucoma. Relative paracentral scotomas and nasal step are usually the earliest signs of glaucomatous functional damage. In definite glaucoma, damage severity can be assessed by various classification systems, such as the methods of Hodapp, Parrish and Anderson and the Advanced Glaucoma Intervention Study (AGIS), and the Glaucoma Staging System. Progression can be analyzed using different approaches including the clinical judgment, defect classification systems, trend analysis, and event analysis. When standard automated perimetry is within normal limits in a subject with a suspect glaucoma, various nonconventional VF testing techniques can be used in order to detect the first signs of functional damage. These techniques include short-wavelength automated perimetry, flicker automated perimetry, frequency doubling technology, pulsar perimetry, and other still experimental methods. It should, however, be remembered that VF testing, even if automated, is a psychophysical test with physiologic short- and long-term fluctuations and possible artifacts.

Visual field (VF) examination is still a fundamental tool in glaucoma diagnosis and follow-up. It is a mandatory test to confirm the presence of VF defects in a patient with suspect glaucoma, to quantify the severity of functional damage, and to assess the progression of the disease. Automated white-on-white static perimetry is currently the gold standard for a reliable VF test (standard automated perimetry). The test programs most used today in glaucoma are the 30-2 Humphrey (or the 24-2), using Swedish interactive thresholding algorithm (SITA) standard, or the Octopus G programs (or G1X), with full threshold or dynamic strategy (fig. 1).

In the presence of very advanced VF loss with a threatened fixation point, the assessment of sensitivity in the central area of remnant vision is of utmost importance. In these cases, special patterns that assess sensitivity in the 10° central area with a denser grid of test points (HFA 10-2 or Octopus M1) should be used (fig. 2).

VF defects in chronic glaucoma include [1]:
1 widespread sensitivity depression (a very aspecific finding, often due to a cataract or media opacities);

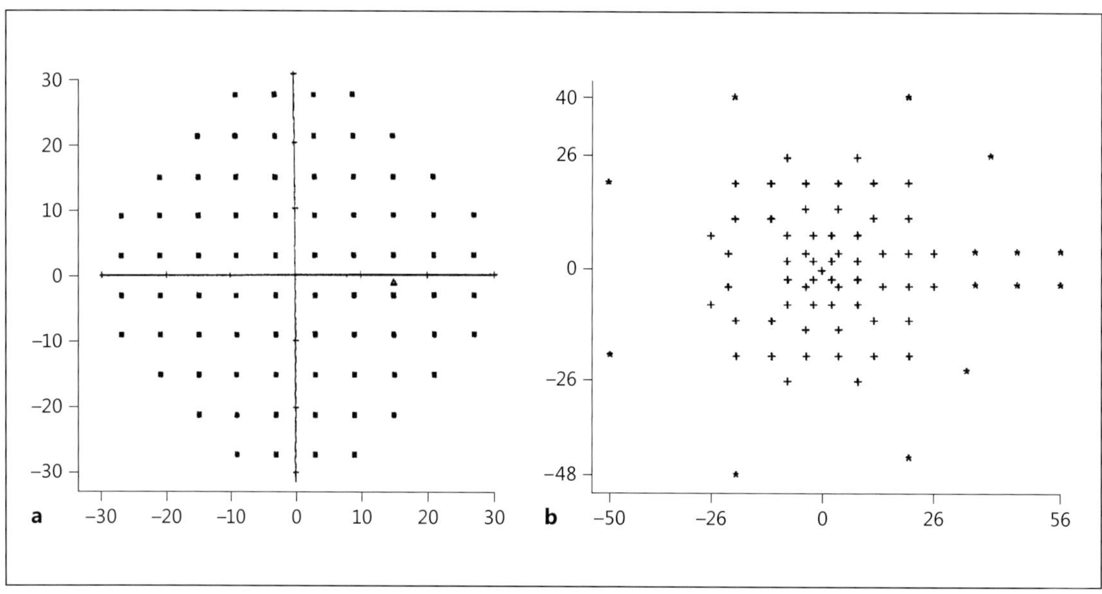

Fig. 1. a Program 30-2 Humphrey (76 points). b Program G1 Octopus (59 central points + 14 peripheral points).

2   blind spot enlargement (no longer considered as a sign of early glaucoma damage);
3   Rønne's nasal step (reflects a pathological asymmetry between the retinal sensitivity of the superior and inferior nasal area; fig. 3a), and
4   paracentral relative scotomas, with a sensitivity depression in clusters of points located within the central 30° (probably the most characteristic sign of early glaucomatous functional loss; fig. 3b).

It is important to remember that a defect should be considered as significant only if it is reproducible in a second, or better even a third, VF test, due to short- and long-term fluctuations that may make the interpretation of VF data challenging and quite difficult [2]. For a correct interpretation of the outcomes of whatever VF test, several points should be considered, which include: (1) test reliability, (2) the presence of artifacts, (3) the presence of significant defects and, if present, the characteristics, shape, and localization of the defects, and (4) the severity of defects.

Before interpreting a VF test, the reliability of the test should be checked looking at the number or percentage of fixation losses, the reliability indices (false-positive and false-negative errors), and the warning messages supplied by some devices (fig. 4).

A nonreliable VF test should not be interpreted; it must be chucked out and redone.

The artifacts, such as those caused by the upper lid, the lens holder borders, or a badly positioned corrective lens (fig. 5), are relatively common in perimetry. It is very important to recognize them, avoiding to consider these defects as related to glaucoma.

Another important issue concerns the criteria used to define a VF test as abnormal. The most commonly used issues are those proposed some years ago by Hodapp et al. [3], which take into consideration the pattern standard deviation (PSD <5%), the presence of clusters of 3 or more abnormal points with a p < 5%, one of which with p < 1% within the 30° central field, and a glaucoma hemifield test 'outside normal limits'. It is im-

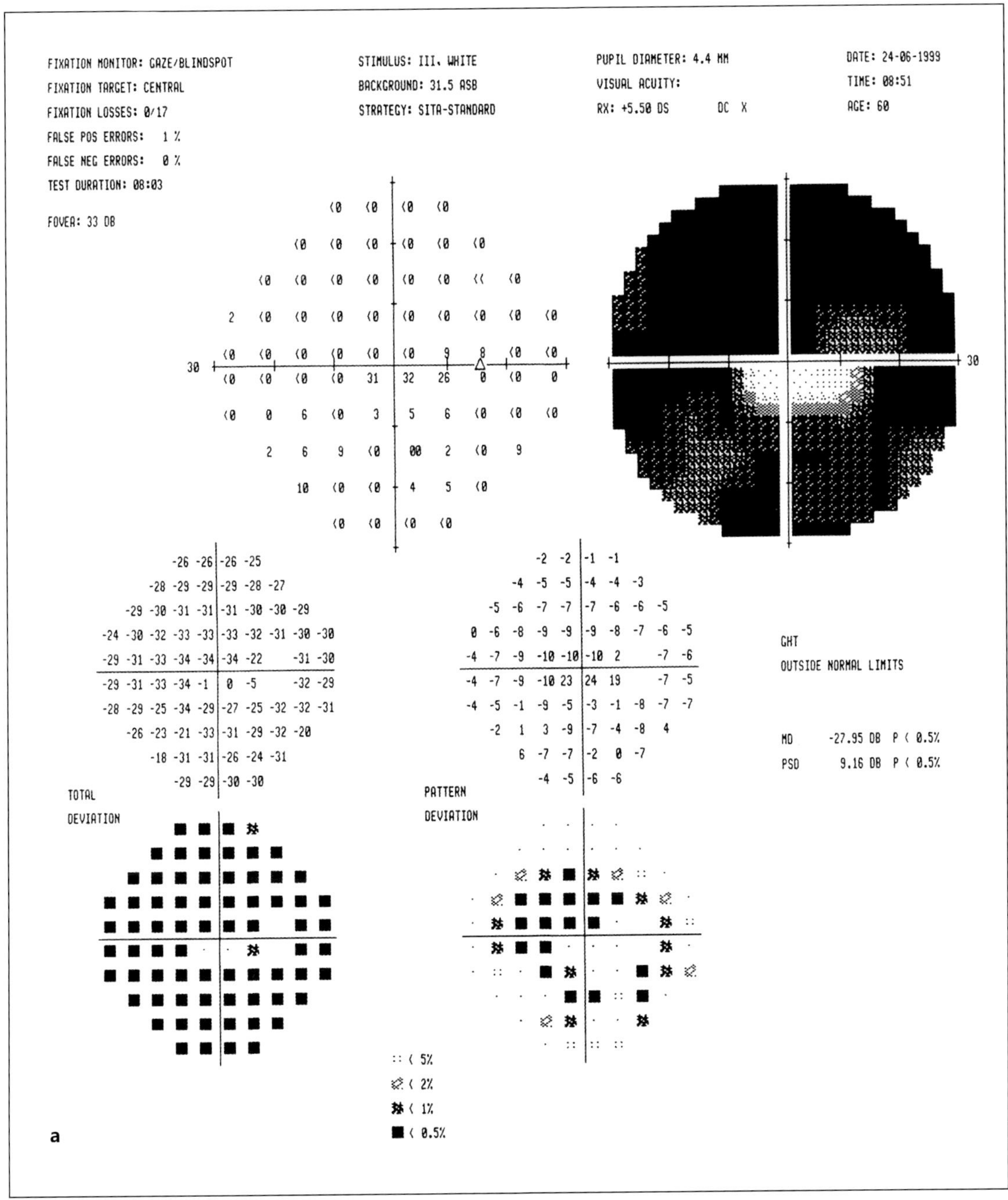

Fig. 2. a Very advanced VF loss examined with the 30-2 test program.

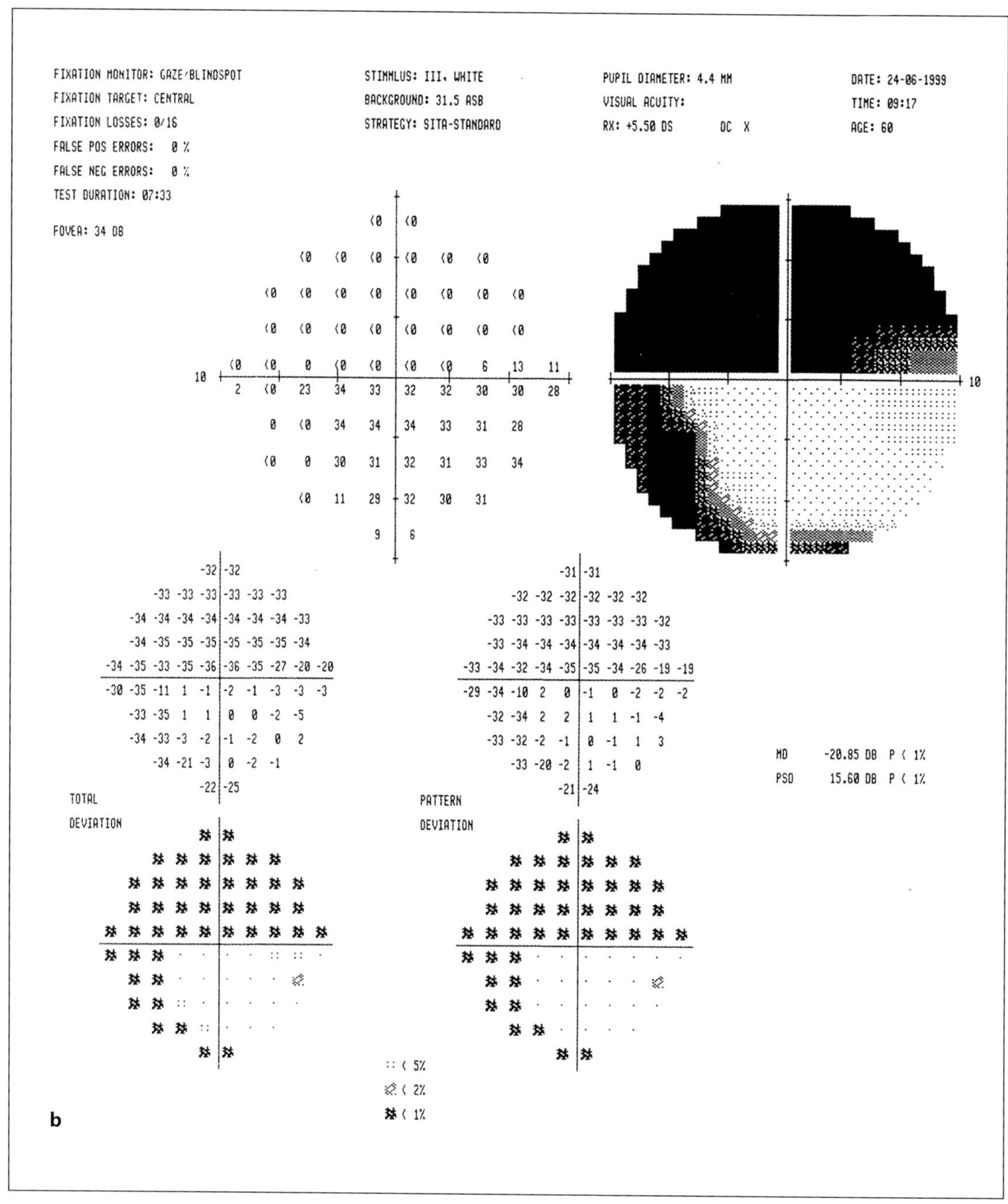

Fig. 2. b Same eye examined with the 10-2 test program.

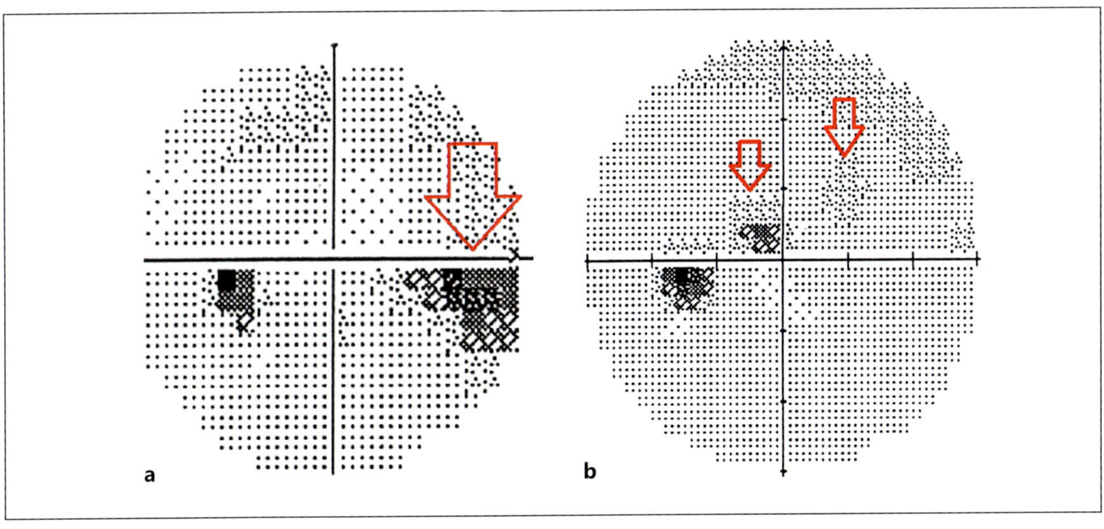

Fig. 3. Rønne's nasal step (**a**) and paracentral relative scotomas (**b**).

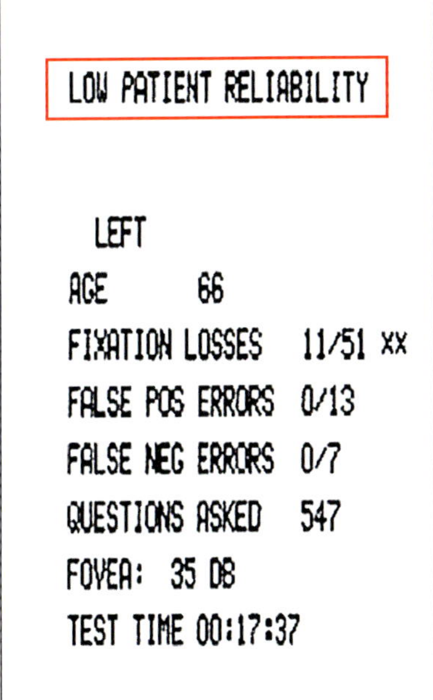

Fig. 4. Reliability indices and warning message (red rectangle).

portant to stress that these alterations should be confirmed in a second test.

If a significant defect, reasonably due to glaucoma, is present, its characteristics should be defined. A defect can be relative, with only a depression of sensitivity, or absolute, with a complete loss of sensitivity (0 dB). It can be generalized, localized, or a mixture of both components. Several methods can be used to distinguish defect type, including the VF indices (VFI), probability maps, cumulative defect curve, better known as Bebie curve, and the Glaucoma Staging System (GSS) (fig. 6–8) [4, 5].

In the presence of a localized defect, its morphology and location should be described (i.e. arcuate, wedge shaped, central, or peripheral).

The classification of glaucomatous VF defect severity is important for several reasons, which include: having homogeneous grouping criteria when perimetry is used to define glaucoma defect severity; being able to adjust therapy on the basis of disease severity; describing VF results in a short and simple format; monitoring disease progression, and providing a common language in clinical and research settings. Several severity classifi-

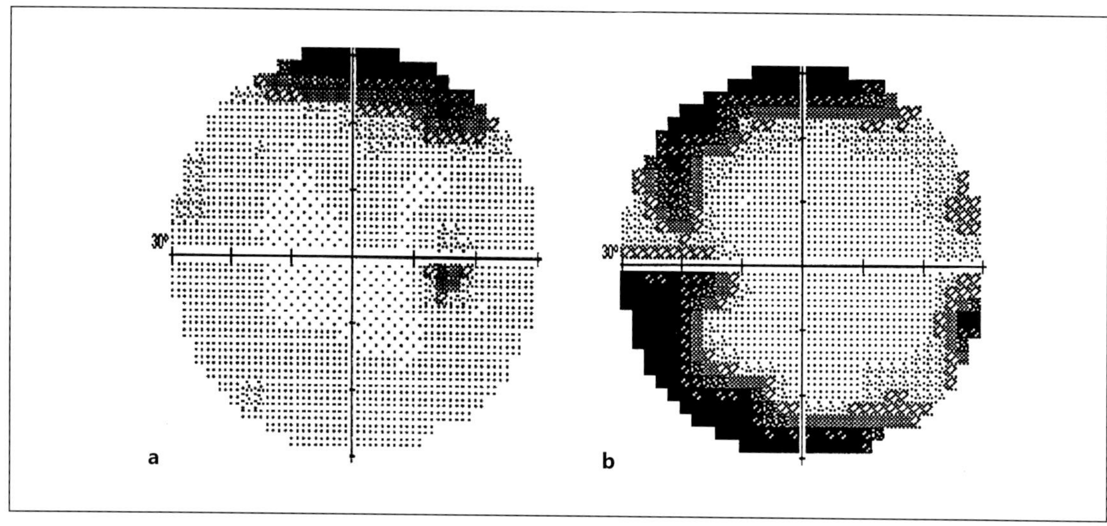

Fig. 5. Superior defect caused by the upper lid (**a**) and ring artifact due to lens holder borders (**b**).

cation methods have been proposed, but none have shown widespread use [6].

The traditional classification method proposed by Aulhorn and Karmeyer in 1977 was based on a large sample of glaucomatous patients tested with the manual Tübingen perimeter; VF defects are divided into 5 stages based on defect morphology and extension (fig. 9).

In 1993, Hodapp et al. [3] proposed a classification method that takes 2 criteria into consideration: (1) overall extent of damage based on both the mean deviation (MD) value and the number of defective points in the Humphrey Statpac-2 pattern deviation probability map (30-2 full threshold test) and (2) defect proximity to the fixation point. Mills et al. [7] recently proposed a new classification method divided into 6 stages, which appears to be an enhanced version of the former method, even if much more difficult to use.

The Advanced Glaucoma Intervention Study (AGIS) score [8] is based on both the number and depth of adjacent depressed test locations in the nasal, upper hemifield and lower hemifield areas. This score is obtained from the total deviation plot of the Humphrey Statpac-2 single field analysis. VF defect severity is divided into 5 stages based on the scores.

The GSS and the more recent GSS 2 is a classification method proposed by Brusini [4] and Brusini and Filacorda [5] which uses MD and corrected PSD/corrected loss variance values (from either the 30-2/24-2 Zeiss-Humphrey tests or the G1/G1X/G2 Octopus programs) plotted on an x-y coordinate diagram (fig. 10).

VF defects are divided in 7 different stages by curvilinear lines, ranging from stage 0 (normal VF) to stage 5 (severe loss, with only small remnants of sensitivity remaining). Moreover, VF defects are subdivided into 3 groups by two oblique straight lines: generalized VF defects are found in the upper right portion of the chart; mixed defects in the center, and localized defects in the lower left portion.

The advances and technological updates over the last 20 years have led standard automated perimetry to be irreplaceable for a precise quantification of the functional glaucomatous damage and for an adequate follow-up in these patients. Standard automated perimetry does, however,

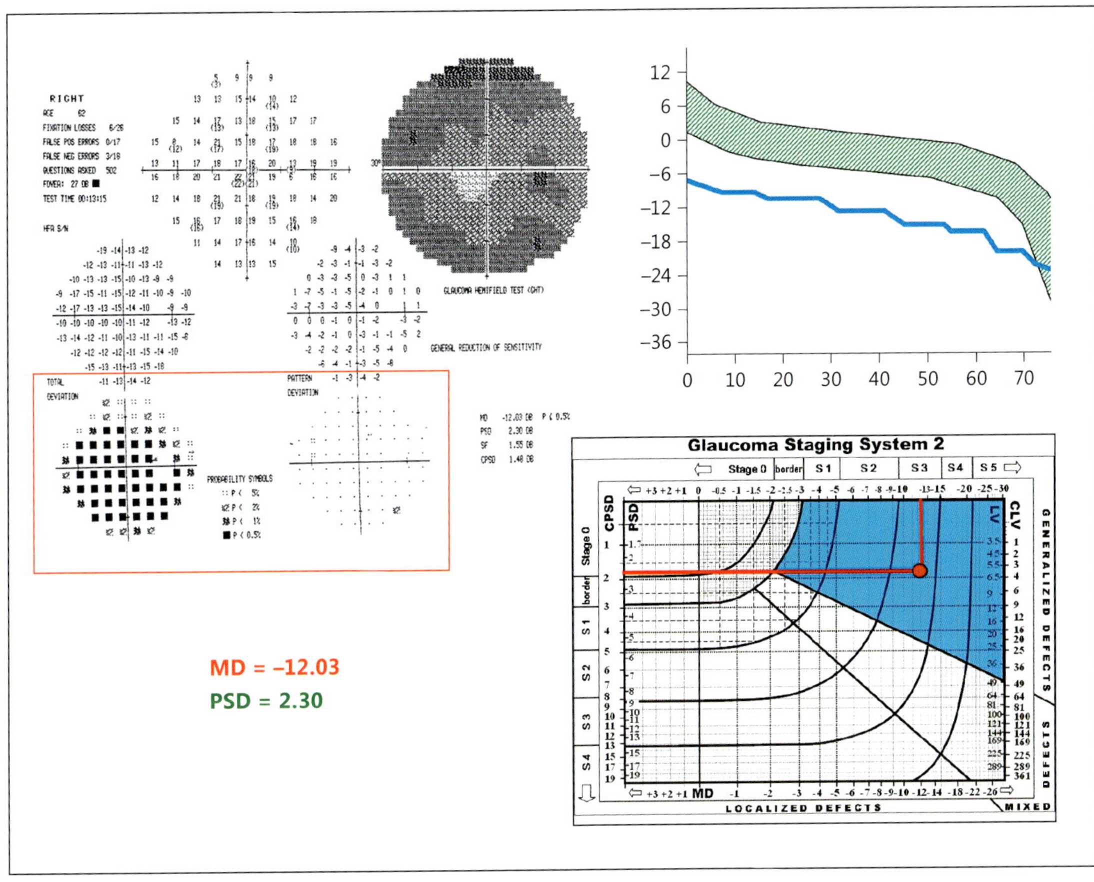

Fig. 6. Purely generalized defect: MD is outside normal limits with a normal PSD; all points in the total deviation map are abnormal, whereas the pattern deviation map looks normal (red rectangle). The Bebie curve (upper right corner) shows a diffuse depression of the line (in blue); this defect is located in the upper section of the GSS 2 ('generalized defects').

have some drawbacks, such as frequent artifacts, subjectivity, threshold fluctuations, and limited sensitivity in detecting very early glaucomatous damage. In order to overcome these drawbacks, numerous nonconventional VF testing methods have been developed in the past 30 years [9]. The most interesting techniques amongst these are listed in the following:

1 Short-wavelength automated perimetry, which utilizes a blue stimulus projected on a high-luminance yellow background in order to specifically test a degree of pure S-cone pathway, along with the small bistratified ganglion cells [10, 11]. For a number of reasons (quite long and fatiguing test, high interindividual variability, and strong influence of lens opacities), short-wavelength automated perimetry has currently a very limited interest in day-to-day clinical practice [12].

2 Flicker automated perimetry measures the critical fusion frequency (number of flickering stimuli/second at which the light does not appear to flash). It selectively analyzes the $M\gamma$ ganglion cells and the magnocellular system

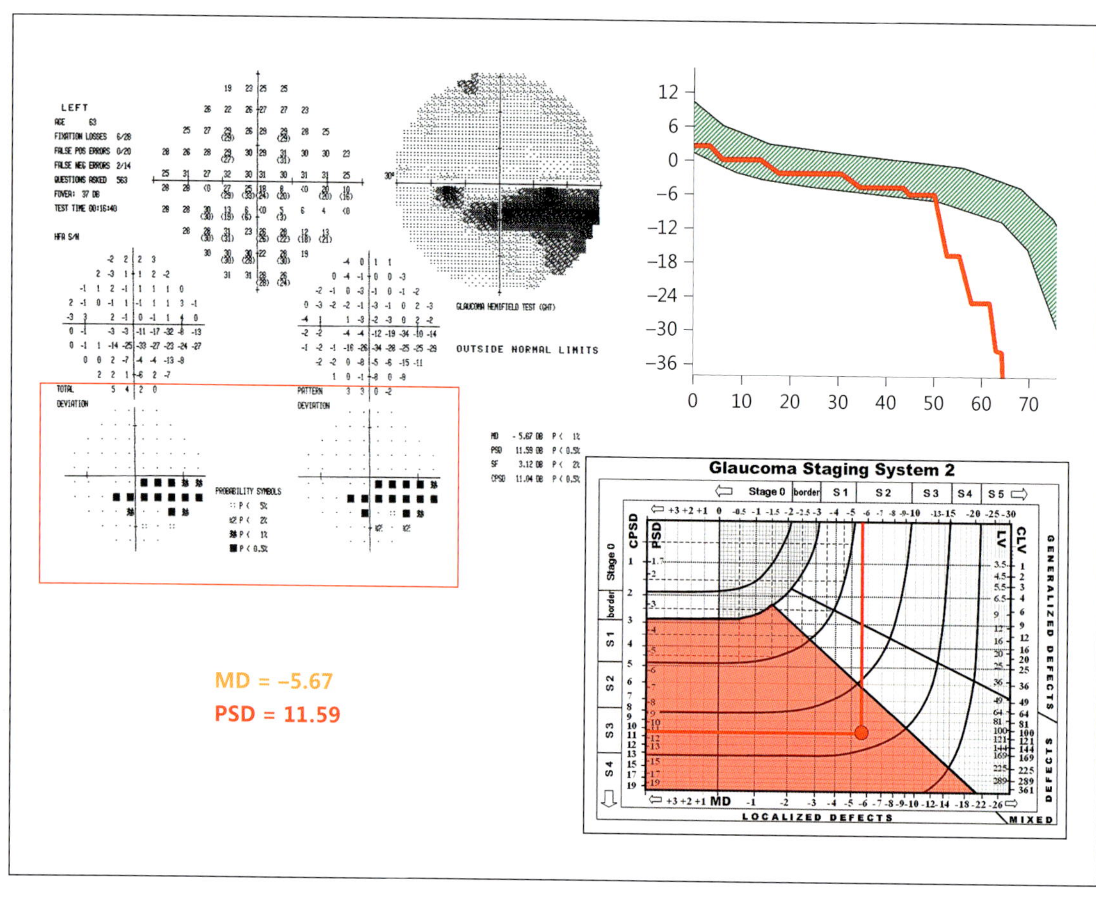

Fig. 7. Localized defect: PSD is more affected than MD; total deviation and pattern deviation maps look very similar, clearly showing the morphology of the defect (red rectangle). The Bebie curve (upper right corner) shows an abrupt fall in the line (in red) in its right part; the defect is located in the lower section of the GSS 2 ('localized defects').

[13]. This technique is quite difficult and tiring for patients and is not of common use.

3 The frequency doubling technology is by far the most widely used nonconventional method of VF testing currently available. This technique selectively analyzes the magnocellular system, which has a very low redundancy (3–5% of all retinal ganglion cells). The test uses stimulus patterns of sinusoid gratings (alternate vertical dark and light bars) with low spatial frequency and high temporal frequency counterphase flicker. Numerous studies [14–16] have claimed that frequency doubling technology has a higher sensitivity in detecting early glaucomatous damage compared to standard perimetry even if more recent researches were not able to confirm these findings.

4 Pulsar perimetry: a round stimulus composed of pulsating concentric rings with different contrast is shown to assess the magnocellular system. A fast strategy is used in order to shorten the test time. The preliminary results seem to be interesting [17].

A very important issue in managing patients with chronic glaucoma is the follow-up of functional damage [18].

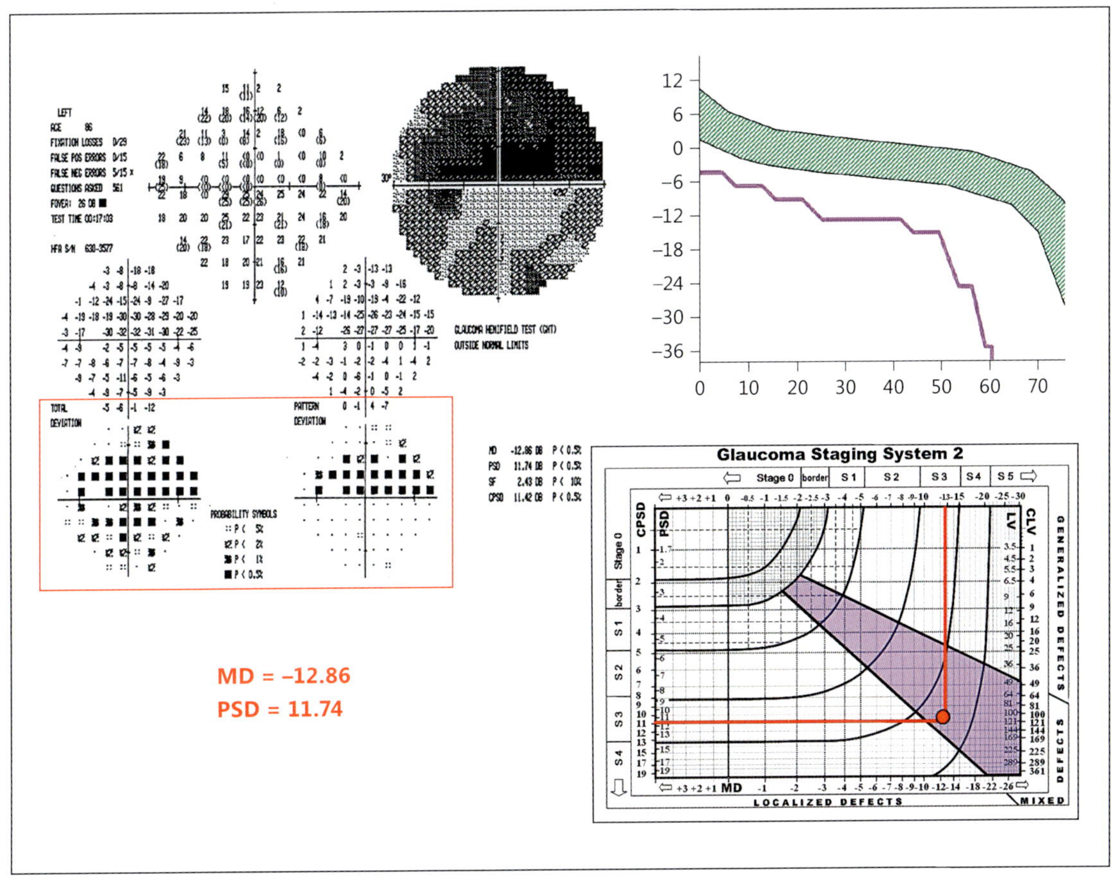

Fig. 8. Mixed defect: both MD and PSD are outside normal limits; probability maps are both abnormal, but the total deviation is more affected than the pattern deviation map (red rectangle). The Bebie curve (upper right corner) shows the two components of the defect (in violet); the defect is located in the middle section of the GSS 2 ('mixed defects').

It is rather pointless to spend vast amounts of resources and time in the diagnostic phases unless proper treatment and careful follow-ups are not continued throughout this chronic disease. It is also of utmost importance to assess the rate of disease progression in each patient in order to properly determine how aggressive treatment should be, which ought to be based on damage severity, rate of ganglion cell loss, and patient life expectancy.

To fully assess glaucomatous progression, both the structural and the functional damage need to be considered. In early diagnosis of the disease, morphological alterations in the optic disk or retinal nerve fiber layer can precede VF defects or, even if occurring quite rarely, vice versa. The same holds true when monitoring progression, in that structural damage worsening can often be seen before corresponding VF defect progression; however, the opposite can also occur at times [19].

Albeit modern imaging technological advances, VF assessment is still considered to be the best method to monitor glaucomatous progression in patients with evident functional damage.

Functional defect progression is most commonly seen as a deepening of a scotoma, followed

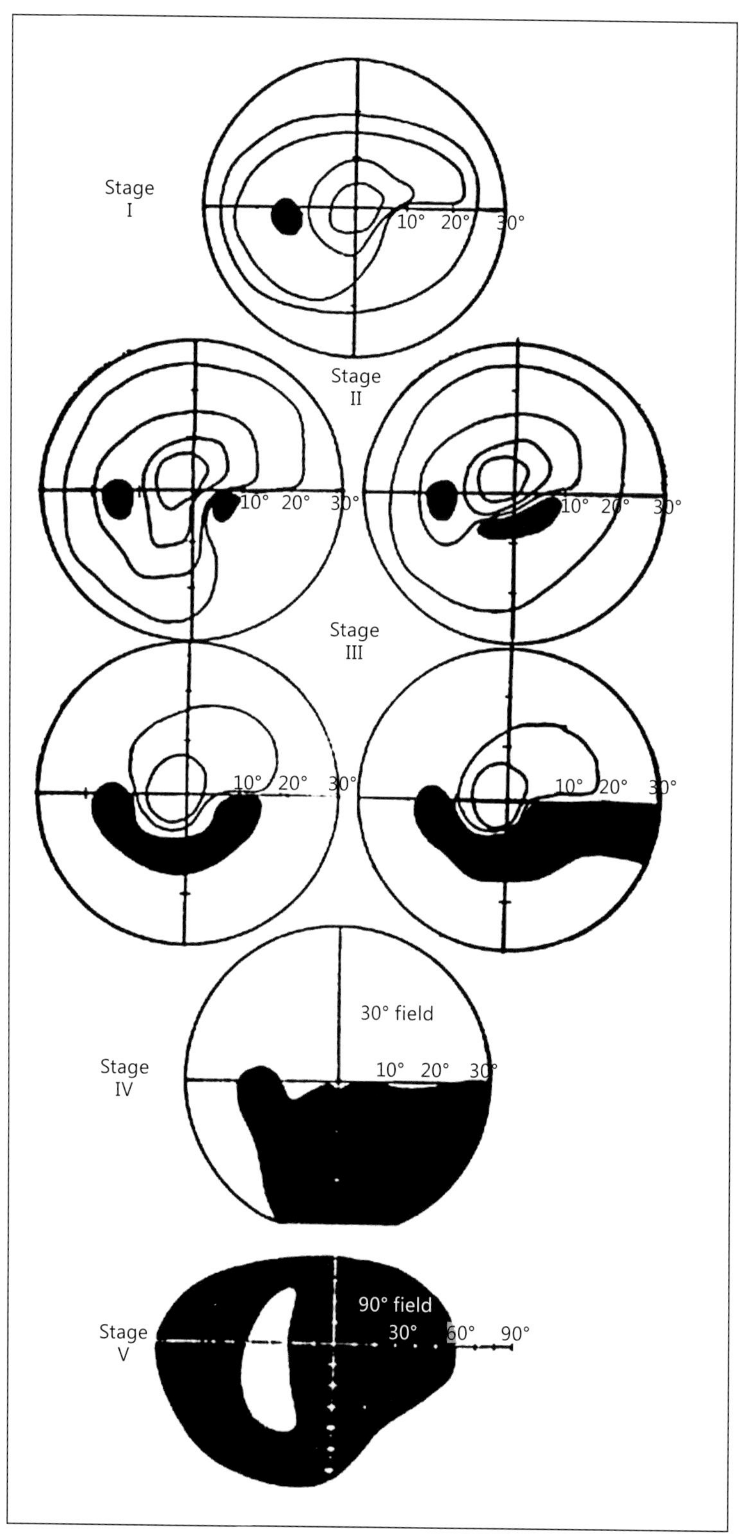

Fig. 9. Aulhorn and Karmeyer's 5-stage classification method.

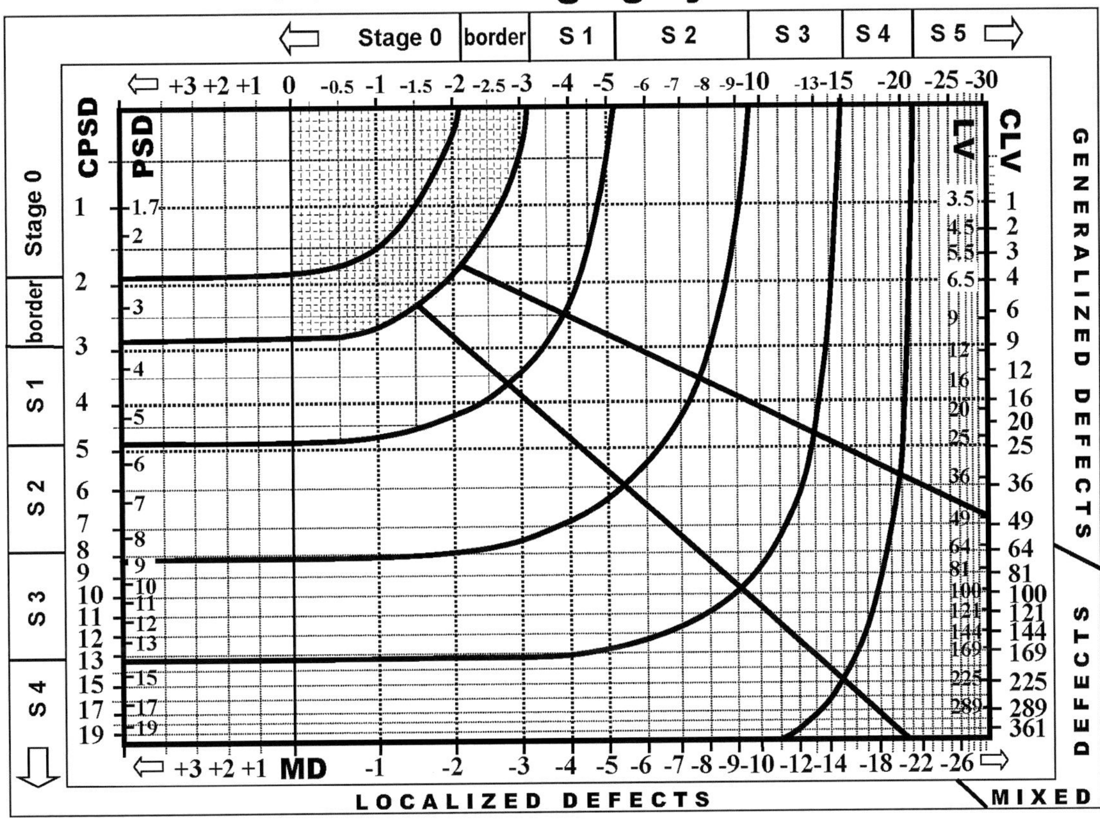

Fig. 10. The GSS 2.

by defect enlargement, and less commonly by the formation of new scotomas. Progressive diffuse sensitivity depression is usually related to cataract and hardly ever strictly due to glaucoma. Full-threshold tests or, even better, SITA standard strategy (i.e. Zeiss-Humphrey 30-2/24-2 or Octopus G1/G2) should always be the preferred method of choice. It is of utmost importance in monitoring glaucomatous patients to have an accurate and reliable VF baseline, thus taking possible artifacts, learning and fatigue effects, and long-term fluctuations into account. The trend to progression should always include the assessment of several VF (at least 5–7) over time. Tests that show significant variations in previous results should always be repeated for confirmation within a short period of time.

Different methods can be used to monitor functional glaucomatous progression over time [20], which include: (1) clinical judgment, (2) classification systems, (3) trend analysis, and (4) event analysis.

Clinical judgment is based on the simple observation of a sequential series of VF tests. It is easy to perform, highly flexible, and takes clinical reasoning and know-how into account. It is, however, subjective and strictly based on the clinician's experience, and thus interobserver variability tends to be quite high.

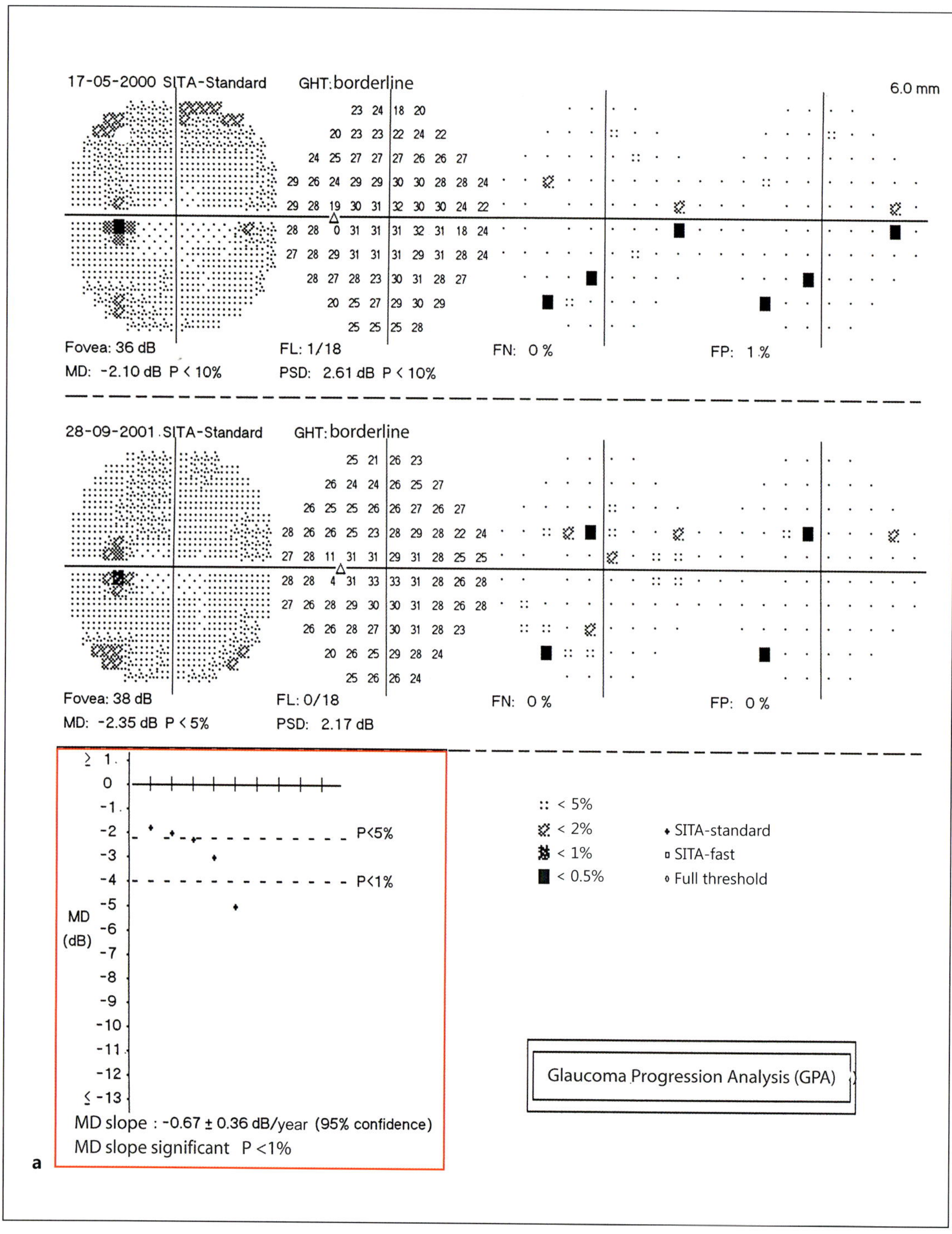

Fig. 11. a GPA program: regression analysis of MD (red rectangle) shows a significant worsening over time. FL = Fixation losses; FN = false negative; FP = false positive.

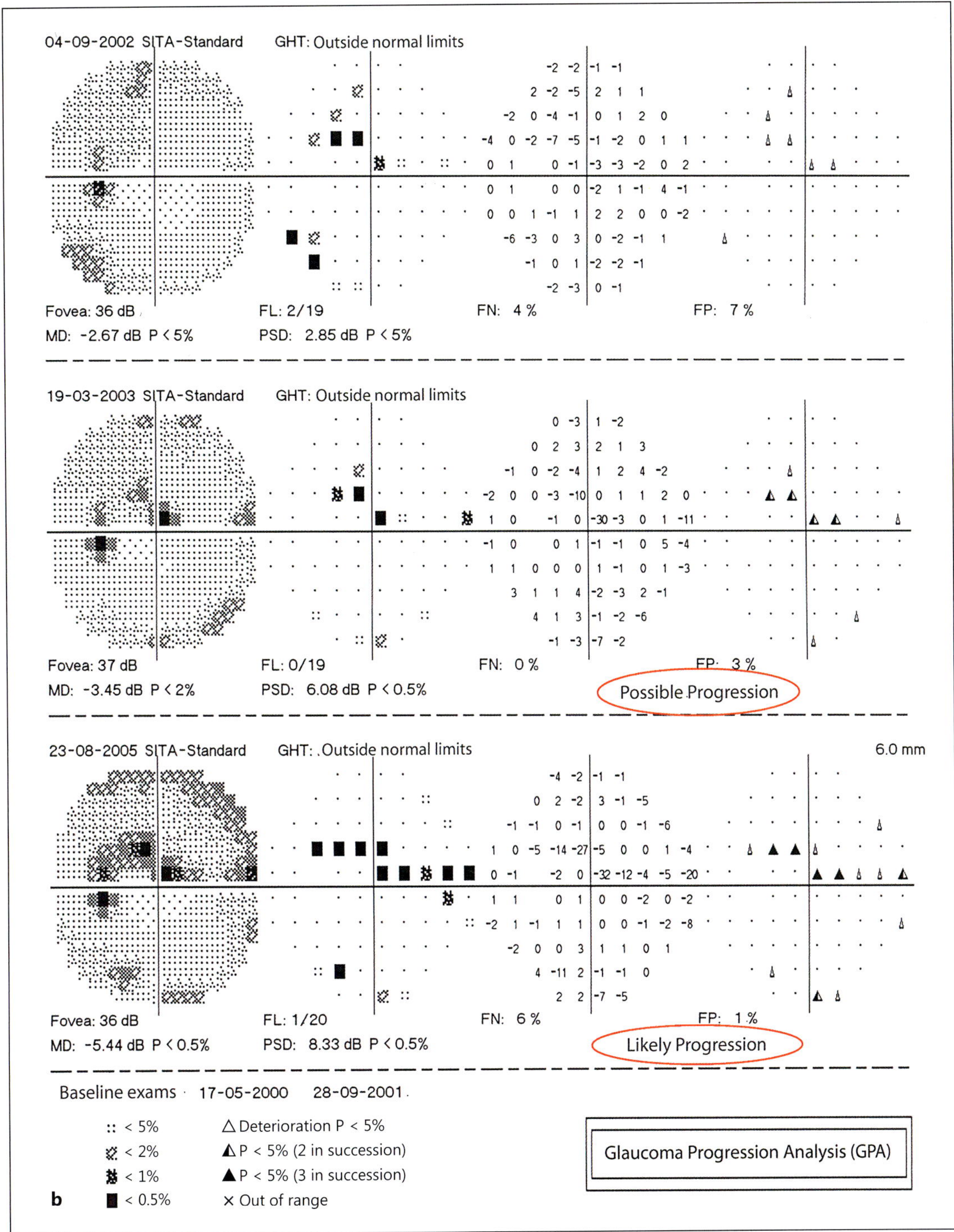

Fig. 11. b GPA alert (red ovals) flags the 4th VF as 'possible progression' and the 5th as 'likely progression', based on the reproducible sensitivity worsening found in more than 3 points. FL = Fixation losses; FN = false negative; FP = false positive.

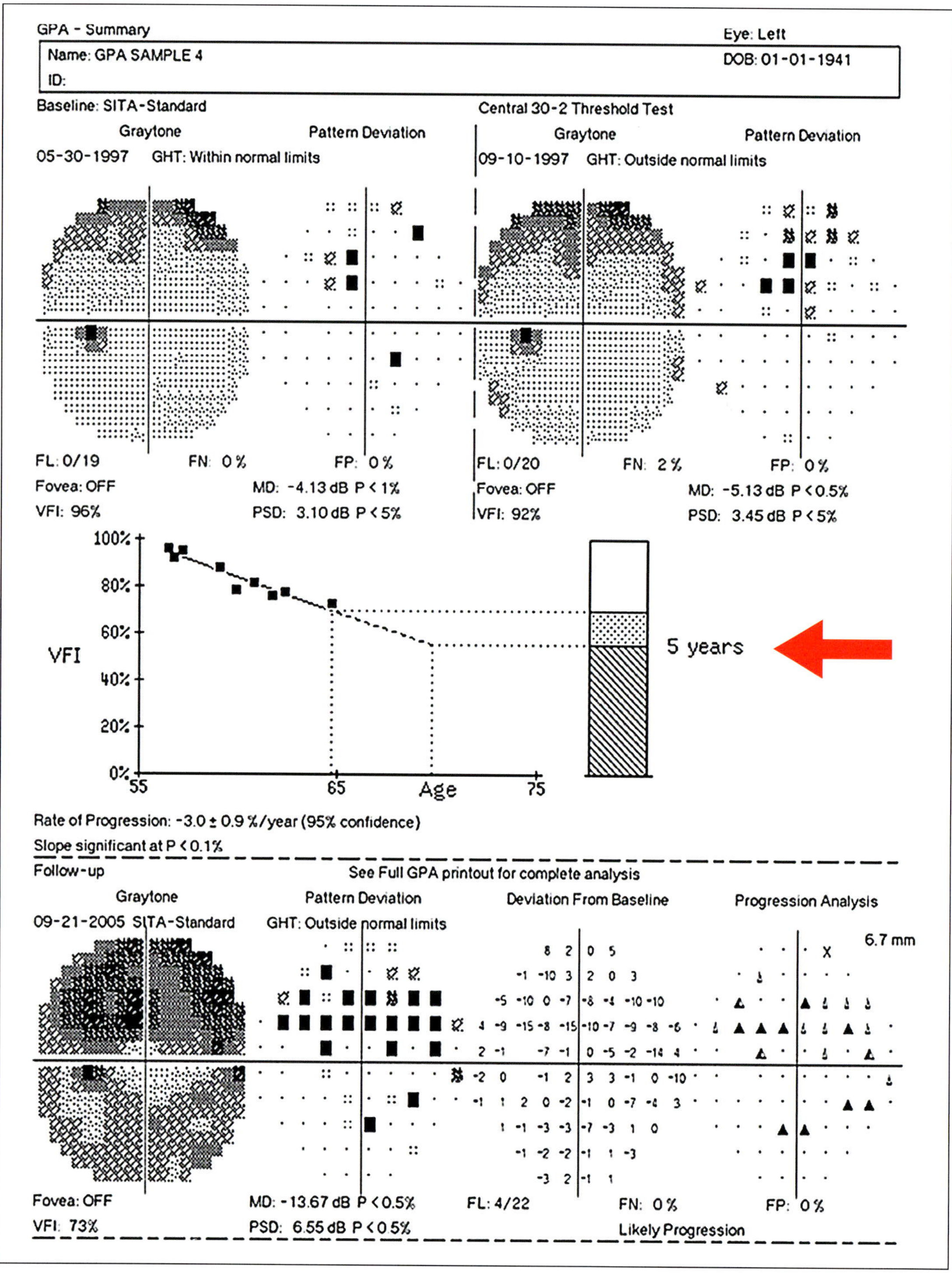

Fig. 12. GPA 2. The VFI bar that shows the amount of functional loss and the remaining VF part after 5 years (indicated by an arrow). FL = Fixation losses; FN = false negative; FP = false positive.

Defect classification systems have often been utilized in multicenter clinical studies like AGIS and the Collaborative Initial Glaucoma Treatment Study (CIGTS). A score (generally ranging from 0 to 20), which is usually calculated from the total deviation plot values, is used to monitor VF defect progression. Progression is defined as a worsening in score (at least 4 units for AGIS and 3 for CIGTS), which must be confirmed in two consecutive tests. The classification systems are standardized and reproducible, but tend to be rigid, time-consuming tests that lack information on VF defect spatial location and characteristics. The criteria of Hodapp et al. [3] precisely define what changes are needed to define VF defect progression, which can consist of the appearance of a new defect in a previously normal area, deepening of a preexisting defect, expansion of a preexisting scotoma into contiguous points, and increased generalized depression not explained by media opacity or pupil size. It is important to stress that progression must be confirmed.

Trend analysis methods are based on the change in a single VF parameter (i.e. MD) over time. This approach is used in some Zeiss-Humphrey Statpac-2 statistical programs (Glaucoma Change Analysis, Glaucoma Change Probability, or Glaucoma Progression Analysis) (fig. 11a; red rectangle) and in Octopus Peritrend trend (which also considers the loss variance index).

A pointwise linear regression analysis is also available in software like Peridata or Progressor.

Methods based on *event analysis* usually compare the latest VF result with a reference baseline and highlight test points that show significant worsening or improvements in sensitivity. The variations are shown as black or white triangles in the total deviation plot found in the Glaucoma Change Probability program (Zeiss-Humphrey Statpac-2). The Glaucoma Progression Analysis (GPA) and GPA 2 utilize a similar approach and provide a 'GPA alert', flagging results as 'possible' or 'likely progression' when at least 3 points show a significant sensitivity deterioration in 2 or 3 consecutive tests, respectively (fig. 11b; red ovals). Moreover, GPA 2 uses the VFI, which is related to single-point VF sensitivity and is reported as percent of vision. The regression line is extrapolated 5 years in the future to show the possible impact of glaucoma progression on the patient's vision loss (fig. 12).

In closing, it is important to note that whatever method is used to analyze progression, VF data must be considered together with the structural appearance of the optic nerve and other pertinent clinical information. Structural damage may precede functional defects, and, in some cases, other causes besides glaucoma may be involved in progression. Ophthalmologists should also remember that clinically relevant progression, which justifies a more aggressive therapeutic regimen, should only be considered when the change is statistically significant, reproducible, and indicative of glaucomatous damage. It is also important to check always the test parameters used (e.g. program, strategy, and stimulus size), to verify if any changes occurred in the tested eye, and to consider all possible causes of VF changes (artifacts, fatigue, and long-term fluctuations).

References

1 Anderson DR, Patella VM: Automated Static Perimetry, ed 2. St. Louis, Mosby, 1999.

2 Kaiser HJ, Flammer J: Visual Field Atlas. A Guide and Atlas for the Interpretation of Visual Fields. Basel, Buser, 1992.

3 Hodapp E, Parrish RK II, Anderson DR: Clinical Decisions in Glaucoma. St. Louis, CV Mosby, 1993.

4 Brusini P: Clinical use of a new method for visual field damage classification in glaucoma. Eur J Ophthalmol 1996;6:402–407.

5 Brusini P, Filacorda S: Enhanced glaucoma staging system (GSS 2) for classifying functional damage in glaucoma. J Glaucoma 2006;15:40–46.

6 Brusini P, Johnson CA: Staging functional damage in glaucoma: review of different classification methods. Surv Ophthalmol 2007;52:156–179.

7 Mills RP, Budenz DL, Lee PP, Noecker RJ, Walt JG, Siegartel LR, Evans SJ, Doyle JJ: Categorizing the stage of glaucoma from pre-diagnosis to end-stage disease. Am J Ophthalmol 2006;141: 24–30.

8 Advanced Glaucoma Intervention Study. 2. Visual field test scoring and reliability. Ophthalmology 1994;101: 1445–1455.

9 Brusini P, Zeppieri M: New non-conventional visual field testing techniques. Min Oftalmol 2005;47:1–16.

10 Johnson CA, Adams AJ, Casson EJ, Brandt JD: Blue-on-yellow perimetry can predict the development of glaucomatous visual field loss. Arch Ophthalmol 1993;111:640–650.

11 Sample PA, Martinez GA, Weinreb RN: Color visual fields: a five-year prospective study in suspect eyes and eyes with primary open angle glaucoma; in Mills RP (ed): Perimetry Update 1992/1993. Amsterdam, Kugler, 1993, pp 467–473.

12 Wild JM: Short wavelength automated perimetry. Acta Ophthalmol Scand 2001;79:546–559.

13 Matsumoto C, Okuyama S, Iwagaki A, Otori T: Automated flicker perimetry in glaucoma; in Mills RP, Wall M (eds): Perimetry Update 1994/1995. Amsterdam/New York, Kugler, 1995, pp 141–146.

14 Brusini P, Busatto P: Frequency doubling perimetry in glaucoma early diagnosis. Acta Ophthalmol Scand 1998; 76(S227):23–24.

15 Thomas R, Bhat S, Muliyil JP, Parikh R, George R: Frequency doubling perimetry in glaucoma. J Glaucoma 2002;11: 46–50.

16 Brusini P, Salvetat ML, Zeppieri M, Parisi L: Frequency doubling technology perimetry with the Humphrey Matrix 30-2 test. J Glaucoma 2006;15:77–83.

17 Zeppieri M, Brusini P, Parisi L, Johnson CA, Sampaolesi R, Salvetat ML: Pulsar perimetry in diagnosis of early glaucoma. Am J Ophthalmol 2010;149:102–112.

18 Brusini P: Monitoring glaucoma progression. Prog Brain Res 2008;173:59–73.

19 Hudson CJW, Kim LS, Hancock SA, Cunliffe IA, Wild JM: Some dissociating factors in the analysis of structural and functional progressive damage in open-angle glaucoma. Br J Ophthalmol 2007; 91:624–628.

20 Spry PGD, Johnson CA: Identification of progressive glaucomatous visual field loss. Surv Ophthalmol 2002;47:158–173.

Paolo Brusini, MD
Glaucoma Unit, Città di Udine Health Center
Viale Venezia 410
IT–33100 Udine (Italy)
E-Mail brusini@libero.it

Traverso CE, Stalmans I, Topouzis F, Bagnasco L (eds): Glaucoma.
ESASO Course Series. Basel, Karger, 2016, vol 8, pp 25–37 (DOI: 10.1159/000446136)

Clinical Challenges and Priorities in Managing Glaucoma Patients

Fotis Topouzis · Pelagia Kalouda · Christina Keskini

Laboratory of Research and Clinical Applications in Ophthalmology, A' Department of Ophthalmology, Aristotle University of Thessaloniki, AHEPA Hospital, Thessaloniki, Greece

Abstract

There are challenges in managing glaucoma patients and priorities need to be determined. Early in the course of the disease, managing subjects with ocular hypertension (OHT) is a challenge. The risk calculator is a useful guide to decide on early preventive treatment in those with OHT and to recommend treatment in patients at high risk for progression to glaucoma. Moreover, although well-accepted clinical criteria defining glaucomatous optic disk damage contribute to diagnostic accuracy, clinical diagnosis remains subjective relying on qualitative assessment of the optic disk. As a result, even among glaucoma experts, agreement in optic disk assessment is not excellent. In addition, visual field (VF) damage due to glaucoma has recently been associated with quality of life (QoL) measures, although a specific threshold of VF damage beyond which QoL is affected has not been determined yet. On the other hand, risk factors for glaucoma have been identified in major clinical trials, as well as the potential role of setting an individual target in lowering intraocular pressure (IOP). Despite this knowledge, we are not able to predict the rate of VF progression of the individual patient at baseline. In addition, glaucoma progresses at widely different rates among individual patients even within the same glaucoma type. Therefore, monitoring of VF changes is important to be able to detect progression and measure the rate of progression. This would allow the clinician to verify if the target IOP has been chosen correctly and to adjust/reset the target if needed.

Goal of Treatment/Who Should Be Treated

Glaucoma is one of the leading causes of blindness worldwide and presents with significant prevalence in the population. It is therefore essential to accurately define and detect the population that should be treated for glaucoma and to precisely define the goal of our intervention.

It is a fact that the question of whether subjects with ocular hypertension (OHT) have to be treated is a matter of substantial controversy. OHT is defined as an elevated intraocular pressure (IOP; >21 mm Hg) in the absence of glaucoma damage [absence of damage to the optic disk or retinal nerve fiber layer (RNFL) and absence of visual field (VF) defect]. According to large epidemiological studies, the prevalence rates of OHT vary

Table 1. Reported prevalence rates of OHT from large epidemiological studies

Study	Age, years	Race/origin	Prevalence of OHT, %
Beaver Dam Eye Study [1]	≥43	White	4.5
Los Angeles Latino Eye Study [2]	≥40	Hispanic	3.56
Barbados Eye Study [3, 4]	≥40	White	4.6
		Black	18.4
Andhra Pradesh Eye Disease Study [5]	All ages	Indian	0.42
Thessaloniki Eye Study [6]	≥60	White	2.9
Blue Mountains Eye Study [7]	≥50	White	3.7

considerably (table 1), while some of these studies have also reported an age-related increase in OHT prevalence [1–4]. Overall, the prevalence of OHT in the population is significant, and the management of OHT patients poses important challenges to everyday clinical practice.

Elevated IOP is the leading risk factor for the development of glaucoma and the only modifiable risk factor at present [8]. However, the treatment of all OHT individuals is neither medically indicated nor economically justified because of the high prevalence of the condition, the low conversion rate to glaucoma, and the cost, inconvenience, and possible adverse effects of treatment [8]. A useful approach to further understanding the impact of treating all individuals with OHT is the 'number needed to treat' (NNT). NNT indicates how many individuals need to be treated before 1 patient will experience a benefit [9]. According to the Ocular Hypertension Treatment Study (OHTS), the NNT is 19.6, suggesting that IOP-lowering therapy would need to be prescribed to 20 patients with demographics similar to those in the study to prevent progression to glaucoma in 1 patient in the next 5 years [9]. Moreover, for OHT patients, the NNT to prevent 1 patient from progressing to unilateral blindness over a 15-year period is estimated at 83 according to both OHTS and St Lucia Study data [10].

In 2007, a quantitative risk model for the development of primary open-angle glaucoma (POAG) in OHT patients based on data from the OHTS and Early Glaucoma Prevention Study (EGPS) was published. This model can be helpful in deciding on who is at increased risk to develop glaucoma and, therefore, in whom preventive treatment might be justified. Although the aforementioned risk calculator might provide significant help, it is important that clinicians take other factors into consideration beyond the ones included in the risk calculator. A positive family history of glaucoma, pseudoexfoliation syndrome, and cardiovascular disease appeared to be risk factors for developing glaucoma in many studies [11–16]. Furthermore, patient's health, life expectancy, and preferences should always be taken into account in any clinical decision [8].

Besides knowing which subjects are more likely to develop glaucoma and, consequently, may benefit from treatment, it is necessary to determine if there is a 'price to pay' when delaying treatment for OHT. The phase II OHTS aimed to give an answer to this fundamental question. In this study, medication was offered to all participants in the observation group of phase I OHTS while participants in the medication group continued treatment. It was, therefore, possible to compare the cumulative incidence of POAG in subjects of the first group, who were only offered medication during phase II OHTS (median, 7.5 years of observation, then 5.5 years on treatment) with those in the second group, who were treated for the entire duration of OHTS (median, 13.0 years) [17].

The results of the study suggest that delaying treatment had only an impact in the high-risk group (40% conversion rate in those with delayed treatment versus only 28% in those with treatment starting at baseline). The high-risk group was defined based on baseline characteristics and according to the risk calculator. This confirms the appropriateness of using the risk calculator as a guide to decide on early preventive treatment in those with OHT and to recommend treatment only in patients presenting with a high risk for conversion to glaucoma. The necessity of treating high-risk OHT patients was confirmed by the RAND study group [18]. In this study, 1,800 scenarios of glaucoma suspects were created based on a systematic review of the literature regarding potentially important factors to consider when deciding to initiate treatment, including age, life expectancy, IOP, central corneal thickness, cup/disk ratio (CDR), disk size, and family history. An 11-member panel composed of recognized international leaders in the field of glaucoma rated the appropriateness of initiating treatment for glaucoma suspects through a two-round modified Delphi method. The panel rated 587 (33%) scenarios as appropriate, 585 (33%) as uncertain, and 628 (35%) as inappropriate for treatment initiation. The results indicated that values associated with a higher predicted risk of glaucoma [greater IOP, greater CDR, and thinner central corneal thickness (CCT)] are associated with higher mean appropriateness scores, with IOP having greater impact than any other variable on panel decisions. According to the experts' decisions, simple criteria for appropriateness of treatment included IOP >26 mm Hg and a 5-year risk of mortality <90%. Finally, a point system was created for predicting panel ratings of appropriateness for a glaucoma suspect that showed a sensitivity and specificity of 96 and 93%, respectively.

Guidelines

There are many country- or region-specific guidelines for the management of glaucoma. All agree that visual function should be preserved or maintained. The 2014 Guidelines of the European Glaucoma Society (EGS) state: 'The goal of glaucoma treatment is to maintain the patient's visual function and related quality of life, at a sustainable cost. The cost of treatment in terms of inconvenience and side effects as well as financial implications for the individual and society requires careful evaluation. Quality of life is closely linked with visual function and, overall, patients with early to moderate glaucoma damage have good visual function and modest reduction in quality of life, while quality of life is considerably reduced if both eyes have advanced visual function loss' [19]. As such, the aim of glaucoma treatment should be to prevent or to delay progression to the stage of disease which is going to affect the patient's quality of life (QoL). According to the EGS Guidelines, patients who should be treated are those with diagnosed or suspected glaucoma who are:

- Patients at risk of developing functional impairment that will lead to a deterioration in visual function related QoL
- Patients with definitive glaucomatous VF, particularly in patients with progressive disease
- Patients with significant changes in the optic nerve head (ONH) and RNFL characteristic of glaucoma

Definitions of Normal and Glaucoma Subjects

Adopting clear definitions and classifying patients is crucial for management decisions. In the following, clinical profiles of patients with diagnosed and suspected glaucoma, and normal subjects with and without risk factors are outlined comprehensively.

*Definition of Normal Subjects without Risk
Factors for Glaucoma*
- IOP within the statistical range (≤22 mm Hg)
- Normal ONH appearance, normal RNFL, without disk hemorrhage
- Absence of risk factors

*Definition of Normal Subjects with Risk Factors
for Glaucoma*
Ocular hypertension:
- IOP consistently >22 mm Hg in at least 1 eye
- Normal standard automated perimetry on ≥2 VFs
- Normal ONH

Other risk factors:
- Age
- Race
- Thin CCT
- Disk hemorrhage
- Family history of glaucoma
- Myopia >3 diopter
- Exfoliation and pigment dispersion syndrome
- Vascular disease
- Vasospastic disorders
- Sleep apnea
- Metabolic syndrome

*Definition of Patients with Primary Open-Angle
Glaucoma*
POAG is a progressive, chronic optic neuropathy in adults in which IOP and other currently unknown factors contribute to damage and in which, in the absence of other identifiable causes, there is a characteristic, acquired atrophy of the optic nerve and loss of retinal ganglion cells and their axons. This condition is associated with an anterior chamber angle that is open by gonioscopic appearance [20]. In addition, POAG is characterized by the following conditions:
- Adult onset
- Absence of other known explanations (i.e. secondary glaucoma) for a progressive glau-

comatous optic nerve change [e.g. pigment dispersion, pseudoexfoliation (exfoliation syndrome), uveitis, trauma, and corticosteroid use] [20]

Characteristics of glaucomatous optic neuropathy are:
- Glaucomatous changes in the optic disk and RNFL
- Focal thinning of the neuretinal rim, typically between 11 and 1 or between 5 and 7 o'clock (for optic disk)
- Diffuse rim thinning
- Localized or diffuse RNFL loss

Characteristics of a glaucomatous VF defect in standard automated perimetry are:
- A reproducible cluster of ≥3 abnormal test locations with p < 0.05 (at least 1 with p < 0.01) along with abnormal Glaucoma Hemifield Test or pattern standard deviation

Definition of Glaucoma Suspects
A glaucoma suspect is an individual with clinical findings and/or a constellation of risk factors that indicate an increased likelihood of developing POAG [21].

Clinically, a patient is defined as a glaucoma suspect if one or more of the following characteristics are noted in at least one eye in an individual with open anterior chamber angles by gonioscopy:
- Presence of optic disk or RNFL changes suspicious for glaucomatous damage
- VF suspicious for glaucomatous damage in the absence of clinical signs of other optic neuropathies
- Consistently elevated IOP associated with normal appearance of the optic disk and RNFL and with normal VF test results

This definition excludes known secondary causes for open-angle glaucoma, such as pseudoexfoliation (exfoliation syndrome), pigment dispersion, and traumatic angle recession.

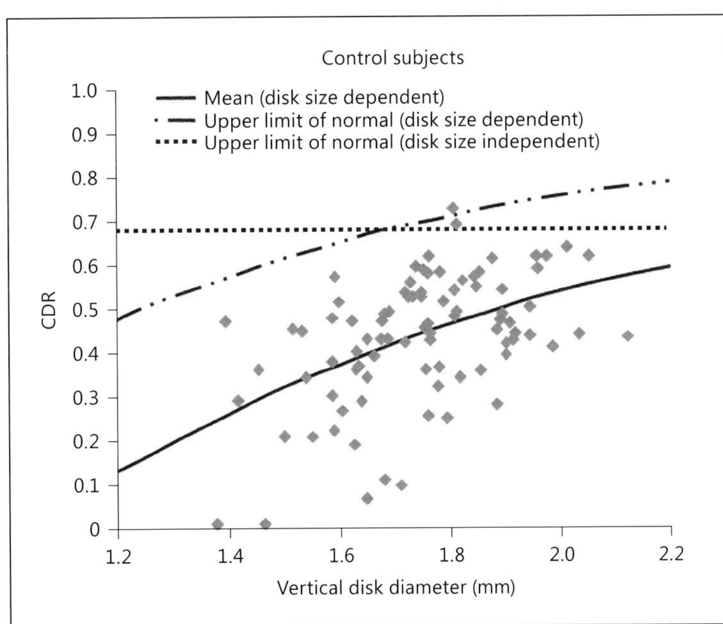

Fig. 1. Plot of vertical CDR against vertical disk diameter in control subjects (adapted from Garway-Heath et al. [24]).

Can We Use the Cup/Disk Ratio as a Criterion to Diagnose Glaucoma?

The assessment of the optic disk is challenging because it is a subjective process that requires the evaluation of several qualitative and quantitative factors as well as familiarity with the range of healthy and glaucomatous optic appearances, and, thus, it is a procedure characterized by significant variation among observers [22]. The difficulty in optic disk assessment was confirmed in 1992 by Varma et al. [23]. In their study, the interobserver agreement of 6 glaucoma experts in estimating vertical CDRs of 75 optic disk photographs was moderate (stereoscopic median weighted $\kappa = 0.67$), emphasizing the need to develop standardized methods for interobserver evaluation of the optic disk in glaucoma.

Garway-Heath et al. [24] investigated whether CDR, in relation to disk diameter, could be an accurate and helpful tool to identify glaucomatous optic neuropathy by evaluating the optic disks of normal subjects, and OHT and glaucoma pa-

tients. Data from control subjects demonstrated the correlation between the vertical disk diameter and CDR. The results showed that as the vertical disk diameter increases so does the CDR. This demonstrates the wide physiological variation in cup size that exists in the normal population (fig. 1). Moreover, although there is an overall increase in CDR in glaucoma patients compared with control subjects (fig. 2), one cannot ignore the fact that there is a considerable overlap in CDR between 'normal' and glaucomatous populations (fig. 3). Consequently, a cutoff identifying all CDRs above a certain level as abnormal would lead to false-negative diagnoses of glaucoma patients in subjects with smaller CDRs but still with established damage (i.e. those with small disks having very small cups at baseline) and to false-positive glaucoma diagnoses in normal subjects presenting large cups (i.e. subjects with large disks).

In our days, percentages of undiagnosed glaucoma remain significantly high, and this seems to be a universal problem. Large-cohort studies in

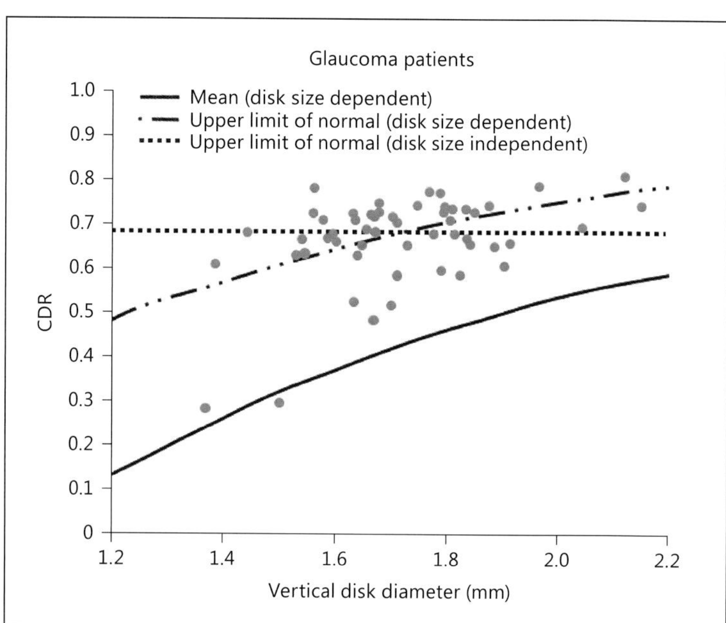

Fig. 2. Plot of vertical CDR against vertical disk diameter in glaucoma patients (adapted from Garway-Heath et al. [24]).

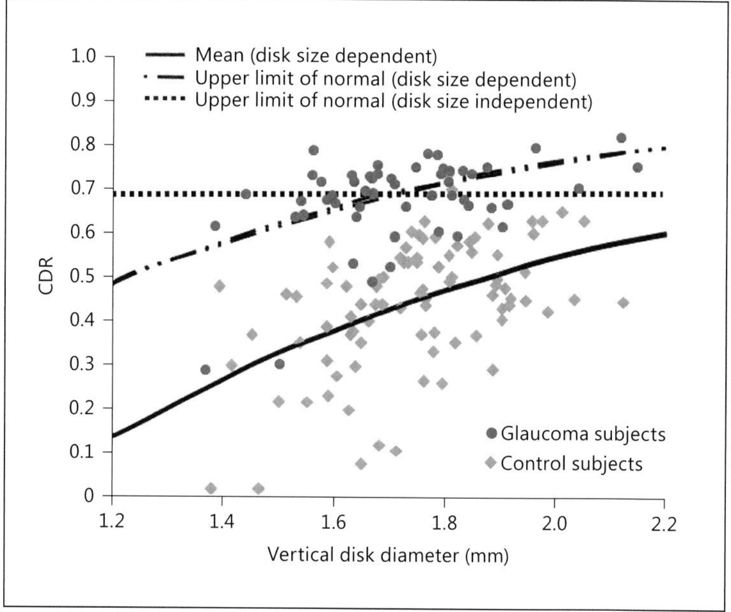

Fig. 3. Plot of vertical CDR against vertical disk diameter in control subjects and glaucoma patients (adapted from Garway-Heath et al. [24]).

different populations around the world suggest that at least half of all glaucoma cases have not been diagnosed, with the percentages for the Blue Mountains Eye study, the Rotterdam Eye Study, and the Baltimore Eye Survey being 51, 53, and 56%, respectively [7, 25, 26]. Even higher rates of undiagnosed glaucoma were reported by the Proyecto VER, the Latino Eye Study, the Egna-Newmarkt Study, and the Aravind Eye Study with percentages reaching 62, >75, 87, and 93%, respectively [2, 27–29]. In the Thessaloniki Eye Study, the percentage of undiagnosed glaucoma was 50.4%, with significant differences between POAG and pseudoexfoliation glaucoma (PEXG) groups (POAG group 57.1%, PEXG group 34.9%) [30]. Interestingly, a smaller CDR was highly associated with an increased likelihood of POAG to be undiagnosed.

There are well-accepted clinical criteria to define glaucomatous optic disk damage (diffuse thinning, focal narrowing, or notching of the optic disk rim) that could make even cases with a relatively small CDR identifiable. Although these criteria contribute to diagnostic accuracy, clinical diagnosis still remains subjective relying on qualitative assessment of the optic disk. As demonstrated by the European Optic Disc Assessment Trial, the mean overall diagnostic accuracy of clinicians was good (80.5%). However, there was still a marked variability in diagnostic accuracy between ophthalmologists [31]. Interestingly, in the aforementioned study, GDx and HRT (Heidelberg retina tomograph) imaging technologies outperformed most clinicians' assessment. Thus, imaging devices providing quantitative assessment of the optic disk and reproducible measurements have established their utility in classifying eyes in the diagnosis of glaucoma.

The Association between Visual Field Damage and Quality of Life

As it was already mentioned, according to EGS Guidelines 'the goal of glaucoma treatment is to maintain the patient's quality of life […], at a sustainable cost' [19]. There is evidence that VF damage is directly related to QoL measures, as it was estimated by the National Eye Institute Visual Functioning Questionnaire, the VF-14 Questionnaire, the Medical Outcomes Study 36-Item Short Form, the Activities of Daily Vision Scale, the Glaucoma Quality of Life-15 Questionnaire, the Medical Outcomes Study 12-item Short-Form Health Survey (SF-12), and the 25-item National Eye Institute Visual Function Questionnaire (NEI-VFQ-25) [32–38]. Although in the Los Angeles Latino Eye Study investigators have shown that there is an impact on QoL even at relatively early stages of glaucoma damage [38], a specific threshold in VF damage beyond which QoL is affected has not been determined yet.

The impact of glaucoma on a patient's QoL is also demonstrated by the fact that VF loss is the primary vision component that increases the risk of hip fractures (hazard ratio 1.9 for men and 1.3 for women) [39, 40]. Moreover, VF reduced to less than 100° of horizontal extent may place patients with peripheral field loss at greater car accident risk [41]. In addition, in patients with glaucoma, deficits in eye-hand coordination correlated with increasing severity of VF defects [42].

Risk Assessment in Glaucoma

Risk factors for the progression from OHT to glaucoma are [43, 44]:
- IOP
- Age
- CCT
- Vertical CDR
- Pattern standard deviation in the VF

Additional risk factors to consider are:
- Exfoliation
- Cardiovascular disease
- Positive family history
- Myopia

Moreover, OHTS [43] revealed the following data for the progression of OHT to POAG:
- Age: 22% increased risk per decade
- IOP: 10% increased risk per 1-mm Hg increase in IOP
- CCT: 71% increased risk per 40-μm decrease in CCT

Study	EMGT [45]	CNTGS [46]	AGIS [47]	OHTS [43]	EGPS [44]
IOP	+	–	+	+	+
Damage	+	–	+	No analysis	No analysis
Age	+	–	+	+	+
Exfoliation	+	No analysis	No analysis	No analysis	+
Disk hemorrhage	+	+	No analysis	+	No analysis

- CDR: 32% increased risk with 0.1 increase in CDR

Risk factors for progression of glaucoma are:
- IOP
- Age
- CCT
- Exfoliation
- Bilateral glaucoma
- Damage at baseline
- Disk hemorrhage
- Race (Afro-American)
- Ocular perfusion pressure

Table 2 presents risk factors for progression identified in major glaucoma clinical trials.

As it was already mentioned, IOP is a well-known risk factor for glaucoma. Studies show that lowering IOP delays the onset of glaucoma. The results of a meta-analysis of nine OHT trials showed a beneficial effect of IOP-lowering therapy [48]. The computed pooled relative risk (RR) of glaucoma conversion was 0.61 (95% CI 0.45–0.83). The RRs were calculated from the cumulative incidence. All studies have a follow-up of up to 5–6 years. The meta-regression model showed that the RR of conversion to glaucoma decreased by 14% with each mm Hg of IOP reduction achieved through therapy.

Apart from its effect on the onset of glaucoma, lowering of IOP also delays the progression of glaucoma. Meta-analyses have been performed in order to reassess the effectiveness of pressure-lowering treatment to delay the progression of manifest open-angle glaucoma [49]. Combining the results from the Early Manifest Glaucoma Trial [45, 50] and the Collaborative Normal-Tension Glaucoma Study Group [51] showed a significant pooled treatment effect of lowering IOP to effectively prevent glaucoma progression (hazard ratio 0.65, 95% CI 0.49–0.87, p = 0.003). The included studies were not significantly heterogeneous ($\chi^2 = 0.13$, p = 0.72).

Target Intraocular Pressure

Target IOP is a useful concept in the practical management of glaucoma patients. It can be described as the highest IOP level that is expected to prevent further glaucomatous damage or that can slow disease progression to a minimum [19]. Target IOP will vary for each patient depending on the:
- IOP level before treatment
- Stage of glaucoma
- Rate of progression (RoP) during follow-up
- Age and life expectancy
- Presence of other risk factors, e.g. exfoliation syndrome

Target pressure must be reassessed and modified depending on the patient's course of the disease. RoP is very important to set or adjust target IOP, but it is not known from the first visit of a patient. Therefore, when first examining a patient, and when the target IOP is firstly set, the other above-described factors are considered (e.g. highest IOP recorded, older age, greater damage,

Table 3. Potential role of IOP lowering in glaucoma management as derived from large clinical trials

Study	Population	IOP reduction	Results
OHTS [52]	OHT	20% IOP reduction	54% reduced progression in treated vs. untreated (4.4 vs. 9.5%) in 5 years' time
EMGT [50]	Early glaucoma	25% IOP reduction	62% progression in untreated vs. 45% in treated in 6 years' time
CIGTS [53]	Early glaucoma	35–48% individualized (target IOP)	No progression in 4–5 years' time
AGIS [54]	Advanced glaucoma	Mean IOP of 12.3 and always <18 mm Hg	No progression in 6 or more years' time
CNTGS [55]	NTG	30% IOP reduction	20% progression in treated vs. 60% in untreated in 5 or more years' time

pseudoexfoliation, or disk hemorrhages). In addition, these factors could also be seen as predictors for faster progression. However, these factors are of limited value in predicting RoP because RoP varies even among patients with the same risk factors.

The role of IOP in glaucoma management was confirmed in large clinical trials (table 3). It has been shown that even a small (1 mm Hg) reduction in IOP could reduce the risk of glaucoma progression by 10% [50].

In general, the guidelines for target IOP according to the Asia-Pacific Glaucoma Society (APGS) (2008) are:

- Glaucoma with high risk for progressive visual loss or visual disability: the target is IOP reduction >40% or 1–2 SD below the population mean (9–12 mm Hg) if safely achievable.
- Glaucoma with moderate risk for visual loss or glaucoma suspect with high risk for visual loss: the target is IOP reduction of at least 30% or the population mean IOP (whichever is lower).
- Glaucoma suspect with moderate risk for visual loss: the patient is monitored or treated depending on the risk and patient preferences. Treatment is necessary if the risk increases. The target is IOP reduction of 20% or to 1 SD above the population mean IOP (whichever is lower). The fellow eye of unilateral glaucoma may require the same target pressure as the affected eye depending on the risk and state.
- Glaucoma suspect with low risk for visual loss: these patients are monitored but not treated.

As already mentioned, target pressure must be reassessed and modified depending on the patient's disease course.

The Concept of Rate of Progression

There are two approaches in analyzing VFs in glaucoma management. Computer-assisted progression can be divided into event- and trend-based analyses.

- Event-based analyses answer the question whether there is disease progression or not by comparing each follow-up examination with baseline.
- Trend-based analyses are primarily designed to determine RoP and show the overall progression of VF defects. They help the practitioner to assess the risk of future visual disability associated with that rate.

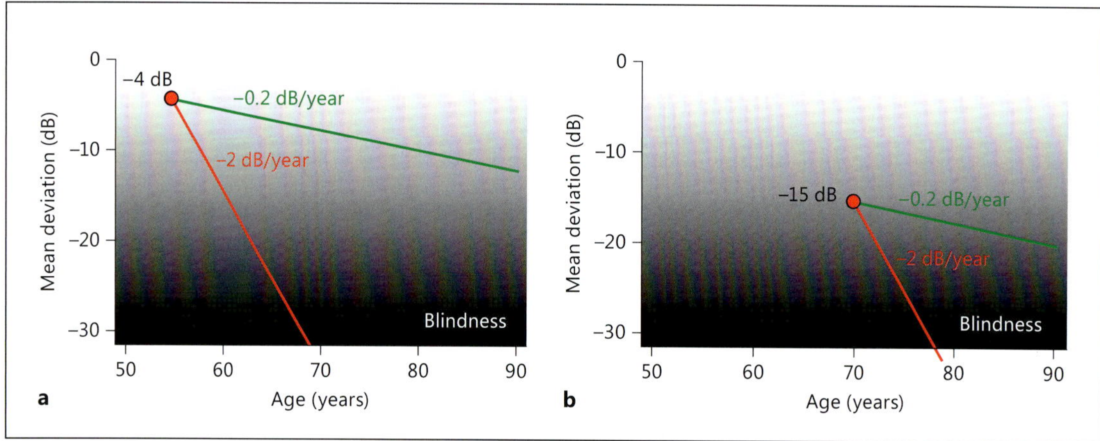

Fig. 4. a A 55-year-old patient with early VF loss (−4 dB) and a rapid RoP (−2 dB/year) can be expected to have visual disability by the age of 70 years (red line). If this patient has a slower RoP (−0.2 dB/year), then severe visual disability may not occur (green line). **b** A 70-year-old patient with moderate stage of VF loss (−15 dB) and a rapid RoP is probably expected to have severe visual damage by the age of 80 years (red line). If this patient has a long life expectancy and a slower RoP, then borderline visual disability may occur in more than 10 years (green line).

Event-based analyses have been used in large randomized controlled glaucoma trials: the Early Manifest Glaucoma Trial (EMGT), Advanced Glaucoma Intervention Study (AGIS), and the Collaborative Initial Glaucoma Treatment Study (CIGTS). With glaucoma change probability maps, all VF tests are compared to baseline consisting of an average of two baseline tests.

Eyes that show deterioration in at least 3 test point locations are flagged as possibly progressing if the finding is repeated in 2 consecutive tests and likely progressing if the finding is confirmed in 3 consecutive tests.

Trend-based analyses are part of Humphrey and Octopus software (EyeSuite) and are more appropriate for clinical practice. Trend-based progression will display linear regression analysis of the VF index. If the tests span ≥2 years, the software will plot a future prediction of progression.

RoP is variable among patients from 0 to up to 2.5–3 dB/year [exfoliative glaucoma (EMGT)]. The clinical significance of RoP estimation as provided by trend-based analysis is highlighted in figure 4.

Table 4. Number of VF examinations required in order to identify progression (adapted from Chauhan et al. [58])

RoP	VF examinations, n/year		
	2 years	3 years	5 years
−0.5 dB/year	7	5	3
−1.0 dB/year	5	3	2
−2.0 dB/year	3	2	1

Considering VF progression among different untreated glaucoma subtypes, the EMGT provides prospective natural history data on progression of glaucomatous field defects in 3 of the most common glaucoma types, including high-tension glaucoma (HTG), normal-tension glaucoma (NTG), and PEXG [56]. In this EMGT report, 118 patients from the observation arm who were followed for at least 6 years without treatment or progressed within 6 years participated in the study. Data were only included until the patient progressed, because therapy could be introduced at that time point. RoP followed the same pattern, but differed significantly among the three subgroups, with PEXG progressing considerably faster than HTG, and NTG progressing at the lowest rate. More specifically, median time to progression was 42.8 months for the total group, was shortest for PEXG (19.5 months), longer for HTG (44.8 months), and even longer for NTG (61.1 months). The median RoP for the overall group was –0.40 dB/year. Median rates were –0.46 dB/year for HTG, –0.22 dB/year for NTG, and –1.13 dB/year for PEXG. Mean rates were considerably higher than medians: –1.08 dB/year overall, –1.31 in HTG, –0.36 in NTG, and –3.13 in PEXG. Differences in median visual function progression rates among groups were statistically significant.

Prospective natural history data have also been reported in patients with NTG participants in the Collaborative Normal-Tension Glaucoma Study (CNTGS) [57]. More specifically, a mean progression of –0.39 dB/year has been reported, and 33% of all patients actually progressed. Some NTG cases progressed more rapidly than others. Although in approximately half of the cases localized VF deterioration was confirmed by 7 years, the change was typically small and slow, and often insufficient to measurably affect the mean deviation index.

Detection of Glaucoma Progression

Glaucoma progresses at widely different rates among individual patients within the same glaucoma type. At baseline, RoP cannot be predicted but can only be measured prospectively at follow-up. The number of VF tests required over 2, 3, and 5 years to detect various progression rates is shown in table 4.

To identify rapid progression of –2 dB/year or more, 6 VF tests in 2 years' time are recommended [58]. However, 6 VF tests in 2 years' time for every glaucoma patient may not be feasible. As a result, clinicians need ways to further individualize their management and to be able to recommend 6 VF tests in 2 years' time to those at lifetime risk to become visually impaired, e.g. suspicion of optic disk change, target IOP not reached or sustained, advanced field damage, pseudoexfoliation, only one seeing eye, increased age, or family history.

In conclusion, it is important to identify VF changes to verify if the target IOP has been chosen correctly and to adjust/reset the target if needed.

References

1 Klein BE, Klein R, Linton KL: Intraocular pressure in an American community. The Beaver Dam Eye Study. Invest Ophthalmol Vis Sci 1992;33:2224–2228.
2 Varma R, Ying-Lai M, Francis BA, Nguyen BB, Deneen J, Wilson MR, et al: Prevalence of open-angle glaucoma and ocular hypertension in Latinos: the Los Angeles Latino Eye Study. Ophthalmology 2004;111:1439–1448.
3 Leske MC, Connell AM, Wu SY, Hyman L, Schachat AP: Distribution of intraocular pressure. The Barbados Eye Study. Arch Ophthalmol 1997;115:1051–1057.
4 Leske MC, Connell AM, Schachat AP, Hyman L: The Barbados Eye Study. Prevalence of open angle glaucoma. Arch Ophthalmol 1994;112:821–829.
5 Dandona L, Dandona R, Srinivas M, Mandal P, John RK, McCarty CA, et al: Open-angle glaucoma in an urban population in southern India: the Andhra Pradesh Eye Disease Study. Ophthalmology 2000;107:1702–1709.
6 Topouzis F, Wilson MR, Harris A, Anastasopoulos E, Yu F, Mavroudis L, et al: Prevalence of open-angle glaucoma in Greece: the Thessaloniki Eye Study. Am J Ophthalmol 2007;144:511–519.
7 Mitchell P, Smith W, Attebo K, Healey PR: Prevalence of open-angle glaucoma in Australia. The Blue Mountains Eye Study. Ophthalmology 1996;103:1661–1669.
8 Gordon MO, Torri V, Miglior S, Beiser JA, Floriani I, Miller JP, et al: Validated prediction model for the development of primary open-angle glaucoma in individuals with ocular hypertension. Ophthalmology 2007;114:10–19.
9 Coleman AL, Singh K, Wilson R, Cioffi GA, Friedman DS, Weinreb RN: Applying an evidence-based approach to the management of patients with ocular hypertension: evaluating and synthesizing published evidence. Am J Ophthalmol 2004;138(3 suppl):S3–S10.
10 Weinreb RN, Friedman DS, Fechtner RD, Cioffi GA, Coleman AL, Girkin CA, et al: Risk assessment in the management of patients with ocular hypertension. Am J Ophthalmol 2004;138:458–467.

11 Leske MC, Connell AM, Wu SY, Hyman LG, Schachat AP: Risk factors for open-angle glaucoma. The Barbados Eye Study. Arch Ophthalmol 1995;113:918–924.

12 Le A, Mukesh BN, McCarty CA, Taylor HR: Risk factors associated with the incidence of open-angle glaucoma: the visual impairment project. Invest Ophthalmol Vis Sci 2003;44:3783–3789.

13 Topouzis F, Coleman AL, Harris A, Jonescu-Cuypers C, Yu F, Mavroudis L, et al: Association of blood pressure status with the optic disk structure in non-glaucoma subjects: the Thessaloniki eye study. Am J Ophthalmol 2006;142:60–67.

14 Miglior S, Torri V, Zeyen T, Pfeiffer N, Vaz JC, Adamsons I: Intercurrent factors associated with the development of open-angle glaucoma in the European Glaucoma Prevention Study. Am J Ophthalmol 2007;144:266–275.

15 Leske MC, Heijl A, Hyman L, Bengtsson B, Dong L, Yang Z: Predictors of long-term progression in the early manifest glaucoma trial. Ophthalmology 2007;114:1965–1972.

16 Topouzis F, Harris A, Wilson MR, Koskosas A, Founti P, Yu F, et al: Increased likelihood of glaucoma at the same screening intraocular pressure in subjects with pseudoexfoliation: the Thessaloniki Eye Study. Am J Ophthalmol 2009;148:606.e1–613.e1.

17 Kass MA, Gordon MO, Gao F, Heuer DK, Higginbotham EJ, Johnson CA, et al: Delaying treatment of ocular hypertension: the Ocular Hypertension Treatment Study. Arch Ophthalmol 2010;128:276–287.

18 Appropriateness of Treating Glaucoma Suspects RAND Study Group: For which glaucoma suspects is it appropriate to initiate treatment? Ophthalmology 2009;116:710–716, 716.e1–82.

19 European Glaucoma Society. Terminology and Guidelines for Glaucoma, ed 4. 2014, http://www.eugs.org/eng/EGS_guidelines4.asp.

20 American Academy of Ophthalmology Glaucoma Panel. Preferred Practice Pattern® Guidelines. Primary Open-Angle Glaucoma. San Francisco, American Academy of Ophthalmology, 2010, www.aao.org/ppp.

21 American Academy of Ophthalmology Glaucoma Panel. Preferred Practice Pattern® Guidelines. Primary Open-Angle Glaucoma Suspect. San Francisco, American Academy of Ophthalmology, 2010, www.aao.org/ppp.

22 Lichter PR: Variability of expert observers in evaluating the optic disc. Trans Am Ophthalmol Soc 1976;74:532–572.

23 Varma R, Steinmann WC, Scott IU: Expert agreement in evaluating the optic disc for glaucoma. Ophthalmology 1992;99:215–221.

24 Garway-Heath DF, Ruben ST, Viswanathan A, Hitchings RA: Vertical cup/disc ratio in relation to optic disc size: its value in the assessment of the glaucoma suspect. Br J Ophthalmol 1998;82:1118–1124.

25 Dielemans I, Vingerling JR, Wolfs RC, Hofman A, Grobbee DE, de Jong PT: The prevalence of primary open-angle glaucoma in a population-based study in The Netherlands. The Rotterdam Study. Ophthalmology 1994;101:1851–1855.

26 Tielsch JM, Katz J, Quigley HA, Javitt JC, Sommer A: Diabetes, intraocular pressure, and primary open-angle glaucoma in the Baltimore Eye Survey. Ophthalmology 1995;102:48–53.

27 Quigley HA, West SK, Rodriguez J, Munoz B, Klein R, Snyder R: The prevalence of glaucoma in a population-based study of Hispanic subjects: Proyecto VER. Arch Ophthalmol 2001;119:1819–1826.

28 Bonomi L, Marchini G, Marraffa M, Bernardi P, De Franco I, Perfetti S, et al: Prevalence of glaucoma and intraocular pressure distribution in a defined population. The Egna-Neumarkt Study. Ophthalmology 1998;105:209–215.

29 Ramakrishnan R, Nirmalan PK, Krishnadas R, Thulasiraj RD, Tielsch JM, Katz J, et al: Glaucoma in a rural population of southern India: the Aravind comprehensive eye survey. Ophthalmology 2003;110:1484–1490.

30 Topouzis F, Coleman AL, Harris A, Koskosas A, Founti P, Gong G, et al: Factors associated with undiagnosed open-angle glaucoma: the Thessaloniki Eye Study. Am J Ophthalmol 2008;145:327–335.

31 Reus NJ, Lemij HG, Garway-Heath DF, Airaksinen PJ, Anton A, Bron AM, et al: Clinical assessment of stereoscopic optic disc photographs for glaucoma: the European Optic Disc Assessment Trial. Ophthalmology 2010;117:717–723.

32 Gutierrez P, Wilson MR, Johnson C, Gordon M, Cioffi GA, Ritch R, et al: Influence of glaucomatous visual field loss on health-related quality of life. Arch Ophthalmol 1997;115:777–784.

33 Parrish RK 2nd, Gedde SJ, Scott IU, Feuer WJ, Schiffman JC, Mangione CM, et al: Visual function and quality of life among patients with glaucoma. Arch Ophthalmol 1997;115:1447–1455.

34 Sherwood MB, Garcia-Siekavizza A, Meltzer MI, Hebert A, Burns AF, McGorray S: Glaucoma's impact on quality of life and its relation to clinical indicators. A pilot study. Ophthalmology 1998;105:561–566.

35 Jampel HD, Friedman DS, Quigley H, Miller R: Correlation of the binocular visual field with patient assessment of vision. Invest Ophthalmol Vis Sci 2002;43:1059–1067.

36 Nelson P, Aspinall P, Papasouliotis O, Worton B, O'Brien C: Quality of life in glaucoma and its relationship with visual function. J Glaucoma 2003;12:139–150.

37 Hyman LG, Komaroff E, Heijl A, Bengtsson B, Leske MC: Treatment and vision-related quality of life in the early manifest glaucoma trial. Ophthalmology 2005;112:1505–1513.

38 McKean-Cowdin R, Wang Y, Wu J, Azen SP, Varma R: Impact of visual field loss on health-related quality of life in glaucoma: the Los Angeles Latino Eye Study. Ophthalmology 2008;115:941.e1–948.e1.

39 Coleman AL, Stone K, Ewing SK, Nevitt M, Cummings S, Cauley JA, et al: Higher risk of multiple falls among elderly women who lose visual acuity. Ophthalmology 2004;111:857–862.

40 White SC, Atchison KA, Gornbein JA, Nattiv A, Paganini-Hill A, Service SK: Risk factors for fractures in older men and women: the Leisure World Cohort Study. Gend Med 2006;3:110–123.

41 Szlyk JP, Mahler CL, Seiple W, Edward DP, Wilensky JT: Driving performance of glaucoma patients correlates with peripheral visual field loss. J Glaucoma 2005;14:145–150.

42 Kotecha A, O'Leary N, Melmoth D, Grant S, Crabb DP: The functional consequences of glaucoma for eye-hand coordination. Invest Ophthalmol Vis Sci 2009;50:203–213.

43 Gordon MO, Beiser JA, Brandt JD, Heuer DK, Higginbotham EJ, Johnson CA, et al: The Ocular Hypertension Treatment Study: baseline factors that predict the onset of primary open-angle glaucoma. Arch Ophthalmol 2002;120:714–720; discussion 829–830.

44 Miglior S, Pfeiffer N, Torri V, Zeyen T, Cunha-Vaz J, Adamsons I: Predictive factors for open-angle glaucoma among patients with ocular hypertension in the European Glaucoma Prevention Study. Ophthalmology 2007;114:3–9.

45 Leske MC, Heijl A, Hussein M, Bengtsson B, Hyman L, Komaroff E; Early Manifest Glaucoma Trial Group: Factors for glaucoma progression and the effect of treatment: the Early Manifest Glaucoma Trial. Arch Ophthalmol 2003;121: 48–56.

46 Drance S, Anderson DR, Schulzer M: Risk factors for progression of visual field abnormalities in normal-tension glaucoma. Am J Ophthalmol 2001;131: 699–708.

47 Nouri-Mahdavi K, Hoffman D, Coleman AL, Liu G, Li G, Gaasterland D, et al: Predictive factors for glaucomatous visual field progression in the Advanced Glaucoma Intervention Study. Ophthalmology 2004;111:1627–1635.

48 Peeters A, Webers CA, Prins MH, Zeegers MP, Hendrikse F, Schouten JS: Quantifying the effect of intraocular pressure reduction on the occurrence of glaucoma. Acta Ophthalmol 2010;88: 5–11.

49 Maier PC, Funk J, Schwarzer G, Antes G, Falck-Ytter YT: Treatment of ocular hypertension and open angle glaucoma: meta-analysis of randomised controlled trials. BMJ 2005;331:134.

50 Heijl A, Leske MC, Bengtsson B, Hyman L, Bengtsson B, Hussein M: Reduction of intraocular pressure and glaucoma progression: results from the Early Manifest Glaucoma Trial. Arch Ophthalmol 2002;120:1268–1279.

51 The effectiveness of intraocular pressure reduction in the treatment of normal-tension glaucoma. Collaborative Normal-Tension Glaucoma Study Group. Am J Ophthalmol 1998;126:498–505.

52 Kass MA, Heuer DK, Higginbotham EJ, Johnson CA, Keltner JL, Miller JP, et al: The Ocular Hypertension Treatment Study: a randomized trial determines that topical ocular hypotensive medication delays or prevents the onset of primary open-angle glaucoma. Arch Ophthalmol 2002;120:701–713; discussion 829–830.

53 Lichter PR, Musch DC, Gillespie BW, Guire KE, Janz NK, Wren PA, et al: Interim clinical outcomes in the Collaborative Initial Glaucoma Treatment Study comparing initial treatment randomized to medications or surgery. Ophthalmology 2001;108:1943–1953.

54 The Advanced Glaucoma Intervention Study (AGIS): 7. The relationship between control of intraocular pressure and visual field deterioration. The AGIS Investigators. Am J Ophthalmol 2000; 130:429–440.

55 Comparison of glaucomatous progression between untreated patients with normal-tension glaucoma and patients with therapeutically reduced intraocular pressures. Collaborative Normal-Tension Glaucoma Study Group. Am J Ophthalmol 1998;126:487–497.

56 Heijl A, Bengtsson B, Hyman L, Leske MC: Natural history of open-angle glaucoma. Ophthalmology 2009;116:2271–2276.

57 Anderson DR, Drance SM, Schulzer M: Natural history of normal-tension glaucoma. Ophthalmology 2001;108:247–253.

58 Chauhan BC, Garway-Heath DF, Goni FJ, Rossetti L, Bengtsson B, Viswanathan AC, et al: Practical recommendations for measuring rates of visual field change in glaucoma. Br J Ophthalmol 2008;92:569–573.

Fotis Topouzis
Laboratory of Research and Clinical
Applications in Ophthalmology
A' Department of Ophthalmology
Aristotle University of Thessaloniki
AHEPA Hospital, Stilponos Kyriakidi 1
GR–54636 Thessaloniki (Greece)
E-Mail ftopou12@otenet.gr

Traverso CE, Stalmans I, Topouzis F, Bagnasco L (eds): Glaucoma.
ESASO Course Series. Basel, Karger, 2016, vol 8, pp 38–51 (DOI: 10.1159/000446147)

Angle Closure Glaucoma

Alessandro Bagnis · Carlo Enrico Traverso

Clinica Oculistica, Di.N.O.G.M.I. University of Genoa, and IRCCS Azienda Ospedaliera Universitaria San Martino IST, Genoa, Italy

Abstract

Primary angle closure glaucoma (PACG) is a major cause of irreversible blindness in many parts of the world. The prevalence of PACG is highly race dependent. However, although less common than in Asians, PACG is not as rare as originally perceived among racial groups such as Caucasians. Different pathogenetic mechanisms lead to widely different clinical manifestations, and differentiated treatments are required. While patients with acute angle closure attacks present with dramatic symptoms, the chronic form is insidious, and patients often seek medical attention late in the course of the disease.

© 2016 S. Karger AG, Basel

Introduction

Angle closure glaucomas are a group of diverse disorders characterized by the presence of apposition of the iris to the trabecular meshwork (TM). Primary angle closure (PAC) results from crowding of the anterior segment in the absence of any ocular disease able to induce an iridotrabecular contact (ITC) and/or peripheral anterior synechia (PAS) formation like uveitis, iris neovascularization, trauma or surgery. The prevalence of PAC glaucoma (PACG) has been estimated to be approximately 0.4% among European-derived populations over 40 years old, while in other parts of the world the disease is at least as common as primary open angle glaucoma. The natural history of PACG involves some conceptual stages: the ITC may cause mechanical blockage of acqueous outflow causing raised intraocular pressure (IOP), either acute or progressive, together with trabecular dysfunction and PAS formation. The term glaucoma is added if elevated IOP leads to optic nerve damage and loss of visual function. An appropriate assessment of the anterior chamber angle (ACA) is essential for a correct diagnosis along with other ocular features including both lens and iris parameters. Besides gonioscopy, which remains a key diagnostic tool in the detection and management of PACG, newer imaging methods for biometric ACA analysis have been developed in recent years.

Definition and Classification

Over the last decade, growing research interest in PACG has prompted the need to standardize definitions of the various subtypes of the disease since scientific publications on this topic have

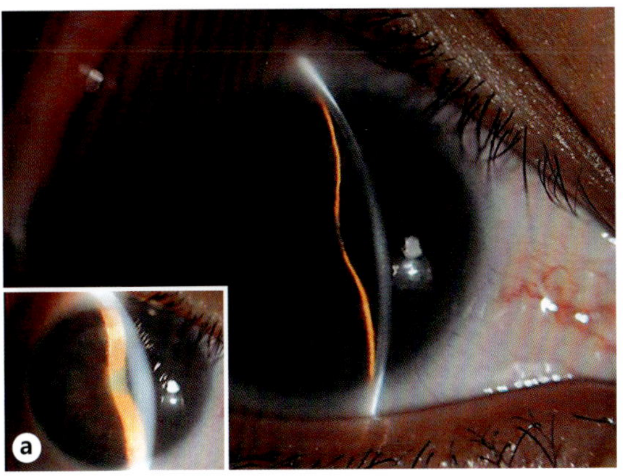
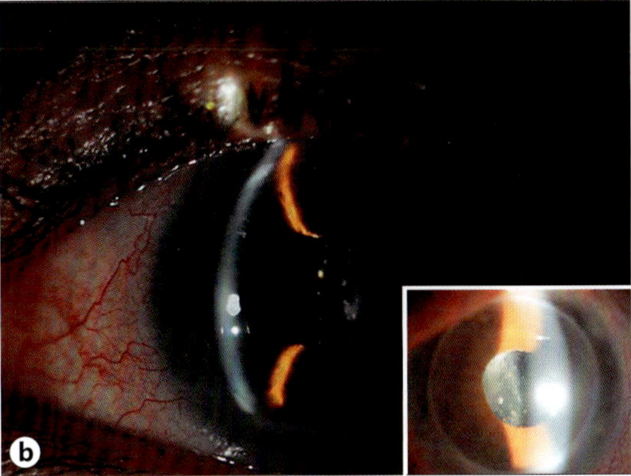

Fig. 1. Secondary angle closure. Iridocyclitis with posterior synechia formation (**a**) and pseudophakic pupillary block (**b**) are typical causes of secondary angle closure with pupillary block. In both cases, with completely different underlying diseases, the aqueous through the pupil is hindered by adhesions that occurred between the pupillary margin and the anterior lens surface (either the crystalline or the intraocular lens). The iris is ballooned forward while the anterior chamber remains deep centrally, assuming the typical appearance of 'iris bombé'.

suffered from the lack of both uniform definition and specific diagnostic criteria. For example, a key recognition has been that an 'acute' attack is an extremely unpleasant and potentially blinding event but not the most relevant manifestation of the disease: the majority of patients suffering severe loss of vision due to angle closure glaucoma (ACG) never experience acute symptoms.

The many clinical entities grouped under ACG are characterized by a variable extent of ITC, which may eventually cause an elevation in IOP and then optic neuropathy.

Staging of Angle Closure
Appositional or synechial closure of the ACA may be due to a number of possible mechanisms. Classically, angle closure is subdivided into two main groups according to the cause [1, 2]:
- *Primary angle closure:* no cause other than anatomical predisposition is identified. ITC causes peripheral anterior synechia (PAS) formation and raised IOP, while no evidence of glaucomatous optic neuropathy is detectable. The term 'glaucoma' is added if glaucomatous optic neuropathy is present: PACG.

Primary angle closure suspect: PAC suspect is defined by the presence of two or more quadrants of ITC, normal IOP, no PAS, and no evidence of glaucomatous optic neuropathy.
- *Secondary angle closure:* a direct causal relationship is found between iris apposition and a specific condition arising from pathological processes in any part of the eye. The pathogenesis of secondary angle closure varies according to the underlying condition (i.e. iris neovascularization, uveitis, or surgery). It is important to identify such situations as the management of these cases is initially directed at controlling the underlying disease (fig. 1). In isometropic eyes, an asymmetry of 0.2 mm (3 standard deviations) of axial anterior chamber depths is suggestive of a secondary pathological process (fig. 1).

Mechanisms of Primary Angle Closure
Focusing the attention on PAC, mechanisms responsible for angle closure are described in terms of anatomical location of obstruction to aqueous flow, successively:
- *At the pupil:* pupillary block is the predominant mechanism in around 75–90% of cases of

PAC [1, 3]. This is an exaggeration of a physiological phenomenon in which the flow of aqueous from the posterior to the anterior chamber is impeded between the anterior surface of the lens and the posterior surface of the iris (through the pupil). The aqueous pressure in the posterior chamber becomes higher than that in the anterior chamber, causing narrowing of the angle and anterior peripheral bowing of the iris, which comes into contact with the TM and/or peripheral cornea. Although the microanatomical basis of pupil block is debated, it is widely believed to be the result of simultaneous activation of both sphincter and dilator pupilla muscles. This produces a resultant force whose vector lies more or less perpendicular to the lens surface when the pupil is in the mid-dilated position [4].

- *At the level of the iris and/or ciliary body:* this group of anterior, non-pupil block mechanisms are the result of variations in iris and ciliary body anatomy and are often referred to under the term 'plateau iris'. These are the result of variations in iris and ciliary body anatomy (i.e. thicker and more anteriorly inserted iris, large or anteriorly positioned ciliary body) resulting in a narrow angle with an angulate profile of the peripheral iris, which is maintained in proximity to the TM or comes into contact with it. Indeed, the typical plateau iris configuration refers to a situation in which the iris plane is flat and the anterior chamber is not shallow axially. These anatomical features predict the failure of laser iridotomy to open an appositionally closed angle: the plateau iris syndrome (which should be differentiated from the 'simple' configuration) is defined as a condition after laser treatment in which a patent iridotomy has removed the relative papillary block, but angle closure recurs without axial shallowing of the anterior chamber [1–4].

- *At the level of the lens:* the anterior surface of the lens marks the depth of the anterior chamber, the most widely known risk factor for angle closure: in PAC patients, the lens is often thicker and more anteriorly positioned than usual, and nuclear sclerotic cataract is a frequent finding [1–4].

Although one mechanism often predominates, each level of block may have a component of each of the levels preceding it, and especially the first two may coexist. Ideally, the aim of PACG treatment is to reduce the IOP by eliminating the underlying pathophysiological mechanism. The appropriate treatment becomes more complex for each level of block as each level may also require the treatment(s) for the lower level(s) [1, 3].

Subtypes of Primary Angle Closure
According to the mode of presentation, PAC has previously been divided into 3 main clinical subtypes [1]:

- *Acute angle closure:* in AAC, a circumferential iris apposition to the TM leads to a rapid and excessive increase in IOP that does not resolve spontaneously.

- *Intermittent angle closure:* intermittent angle closure is similar to AAC but spontaneously resolving.

- *Chronic angle closure:* a permanent synechial closure of any extent is detectable in chronic angle closure.

Primary angle closure suspect: PAC suspect or 'occludable angle' is a clinical assessment with no precise indication to treatment valid for all cases (see also Ocular Manifestations and Diagnosis).

Status after an acute angle closure attack: this refers to typical signs detectable after an AAC attack: patchy iris atrophy, iris torsion, posterior synechiae, poorly reactive/nonreactive pupil, anterior subcapsular or capsular opacities of the lens ('Glaukomflecken'), PAS, or reduced endothelial cell count.

There is debate on whether this approach to classification is useful in determining the prognosis or optimal management [1].

Independently of the specific pathogenetic mechanism(s) determining angle closure, aqueous outflow may be impaired by at least 2 conceptual ways [1, 4]:

- Simple physical obstruction of the TM by the iris. This is probably the precipitating event in symptomatic (acute) angle closure, when a massive/total obstruction of the TM leads to a rapid and dramatic IOP increase. Worth of note, in most of these cases, at least some amount of ITC was *already* present *before* the AAC and did not occur *acutely*: the number of people with ITC far exceeds the number suffering AAC. Indeed, the most commonly identified sign indicating that treatment is required and is expected to be effective is the detection of ITC.
- Irreversible degeneration and damage of the TM either by PAS formation or as a result of long-standing appositional closure. Prolonged appositional ITC may cause the formation of PAS, which may be the result of an episode of AAC or inflammation of any other anterior segment as well. Moreover, prolonged and possibly only intermittent frictional ITC over time is likely to be able to degrade TM structure and function, not necessarily accompanied by PAS formation. Histological data have shown gross changes in TM architecture in both AAC attack and asymptomatic cases. Interestingly, in the second group, such alterations were detectable also in areas where PAS had not formed, suggesting that low-grade ITC may be sufficient to cause TM functional degradation [5].

Prevalence and Incidence

Striking differences in the distribution of PACG by racial groups have been reported in several studies [1–4].

Among Caucasians, the prevalence of angle closure varies between 0.1 and 0.6%, corresponding to 1.60 million people affected by PACG in Europe [6]. Similarly, angle closure is regarded as uncommon in Africa, with a reported prevalence of 0.5% or less. However, the heterogeneity of the continent's population cannot allow generalizations about patterns of the disease: for instance, the prevalence of angle closure in a group of mixed races in Cape Malay was found to be 2.3%. In the USA, it is estimated that about 580,000 people have PACG [1]. Among Asian people, prevalence rates of the disease are higher than in Europe, varying between 0.3 and 4.3%, and PACG is acknowledged as a major cause of ocular morbidity in the Chinese population, where it has been estimated that around 28 million people have narrow angles and 9 million significant angle closure, leading PACG to be responsible for more than 90% of bilateral blindness due to glaucoma. Age- and gender-standardized incidence rates of symptomatic ('acute') angle closure have been reported to range from 4.7 in Finland to 15.5 among Chinese Singaporeans [4]. Although the available data are conflicting and report a prevalence varying between 0.7 and 4.3%, PACG is likely to be significantly more common in India than in Europe as well. However, the highest prevalence rates of the disease have been reported among the Inuit populations (2.2–6.2%) [2, 7].

Differences in pathogenetic mechanisms, symptoms, and severity of visual field damage between different ethnicities have been also reported, with higher visual morbidity in Asians than Caucasians [8, 9].

Risk Factors

Regardless of the ethnic background, which is considered one of the major factors determining susceptibility to PAC, prevalence and incidence increase uniformly with age as a consequence of the lifelong increase in lens volume. Women are affected more often than men, independent of age [10]. One study among Inuits showed a 16% incidence of angle closure over a decade in high-risk suspects, and the vast majority of the incident cases (83%) were women [11]; three quarters (75%) of PACG cases noted in European-derived populations occur in female patients.

A significantly increased risk of angle closure exists in family members of an affected patient: first-degree relatives may have a 1 in 4 risk of a PAC disease requiring treatment, and family screening is vital in these families [1].

The risk of ITC on a 'narrow' angle begins to increase once the angle is ≤20°. In such cases, signs of previous angle closure (i.e. PAS or iris pigment on the TM) should be carefully sought as signs of previous closure. Besides iris apposition/ adhesion to the TM, a hallmark of the most common form of PACG is some degree of pupillary block or increased resistance to transpupillary flow to aqueous humor.

Ocular Biometry and the Lens
Many of the anatomical features characteristic of PACG can be explained by trends in ocular biometry:
- Shallow anterior chamber depth
- Thicker lens and/or increased anterior curvature of the lens
- Anteriorly located lens
- Shorter axial length and increased ratio of the lens thickness to the axial length
- Smaller corneal diameter

The influence of the lens on the etiology of ACG has been well established. Indeed, all the above-mentioned anatomical features characteristic of angle closure are those predisposing to the apposition of the posterior surface of the iris to the anterior surface of the lens, and both position and thickness of the lens determine the depth of the anterior chamber, which is considered the major risk factor for the development of angle closure.

The above-mentioned demographic factors, increasing age and female gender, are both associated with shallower anterior chambers, and people developing angle closure tend to have shallower anterior chambers than the unaffected ones in all populations studied to date.

It has been calculated that two thirds of the anterior chamber depth difference between ACG patients and normal controls is attributable to a more anterior position of the lens and one third to the lens being thicker than normal [4].

At least among Europeans, the lens becomes more steeply curved with advancing age, and there is a close correlation between thickness and anterior curvature of the lens and an inverse correlation between lens curvature and axial length [4].

The Iris
More recently, anterior segment imaging techniques have allowed to assess a range of new angle parameters and have been used to focus on the iris features. Studies using these methods identified the following iris parameters to be associated with angle closure [12]:
- Thickness
- Curvature
- Area
- Volume

Besides *static* anatomical features, the dynamic behavior of intraocular structures, specifically of the iris, has also been advocated as a risk factor for angle closure. Anterior segment (AS)-optical coherence tomography (OCT) studies showed that the iris volume routinely shrinks on pupil dilation, confirming previous data suggesting that the iris might occlude many angles unless the iris volume got somewhat smaller as the pupil enlarges [13]. It has been proposed that the iris loses volume while dilating by a loss of stromal extracellular fluid. Eyes with more compact or water-retentive iris stroma would lose less volume than normal or even increase it by a relative constriction of venous outflow, thus narrowing the angle and predisposing to angle closure [14].

In ACG, like in other complex disorders, all individuals with disease do not share exactly the same set of risk factors, and often different mechanisms may coexist although one predominates. Overall, it is evident that ACG is caused by a combination of smaller eye dimensions and altered dynamic behavior of intraocular structures in most patients.

Typically, the prevalence of PACG is higher in the elderly, hyperopic patients, and PAC is rarely observed in myopic eyes [15, 16]. A decline in the rates of patients with PACG in England during recent years, after a long period of increases in rates of patients undergoing cataract surgery, has been reported [17, 18]. These data support the hypothesis that cataract surgery may reduce the likelihood of PACG and stress the importance of all the predisposing factors mentioned above in its pathogenesis.

Ocular Manifestations and Diagnosis

Signs and Symptoms

As previously mentioned, signs and symptoms of angle closure may vary, depending on the specific pathogenetic mechanism and subtype.

Acute angle closure is characterized by sudden, circumferential iridotrabecular apposition that causes a rapid, severe, and symptomatic rise in IOP. Symptoms include sudden decrease in vision, halos around lights, frontal headache, pain, nausea, and vomiting. Signs detected by slit lamp examination include conjunctival congestion, corneal edema, shallow or flat anterior chamber, and a mild-dilated pupil not reacting to light. IOP is always elevated, often up to 50–70 mm Hg.

Intermittent angle closure (also called subacute angle closure), signs and symptoms are similar but generally milder than during an acute attack and resolution is spontaneous, as the episodes of iridotrabecular apposition are self-limiting.

During *chronic angle closure*, irreversible iridotrabecular adhesion with permanent synechial closure of any extent slowly develops; few or no symptoms are present unless the gradually increasing IOP significantly elevates or advanced visual field damage is present.

The severity of glaucomatous optic nerve damage during PACG is generally proportional to the duration and values of elevated IOP.

Differences in the effects of PACG and primary open-angle glaucoma (POAG) on the optic nerve and visual field have been hypothesized. It would be expected that high IOP lasting for a limited time (i.e. in eyes undergoing AAC attacks) would produce a different alteration in the structure of the optic disk or loss of function than would longer lower levels of IOP, i.e. during chronic ACG (CACG) or POAG. Moreover, it has been proposed that differences between PACG and POAG might relate to differences in the optic disk structure and the susceptibility of retinal ganglion cells to injury. However, no definitive data exist about this topic [19–21].

Usually, both eyes of each patient show similar anatomic features predisposing to an AAC attack or to other forms of PACG.

The *occludable angle* is not an objective finding but rather a clinical judgment as it derives from an overall evaluation in which gonioscopy plays a pivotal role.

Diagnosis

The van Herick Method

Any comprehensive eye examination should include a slit lamp grading of peripheral anterior chamber depth. The van Herick method is based on the use of corneal thickness as a unit measure of the depth of the anterior chamber at the furthest periphery. Based on this system, anterior chamber depth is graded from 0 (iridocorneal contact) to 4 (iridocorneal distance = corneal thickness), with each grade corresponding to a rough indication on the likelihood of angle closure. When the space between iris and corneal endothelium is <1/4 (grade 1), angle closure is likely, when it is ≥1/4 and <1/2

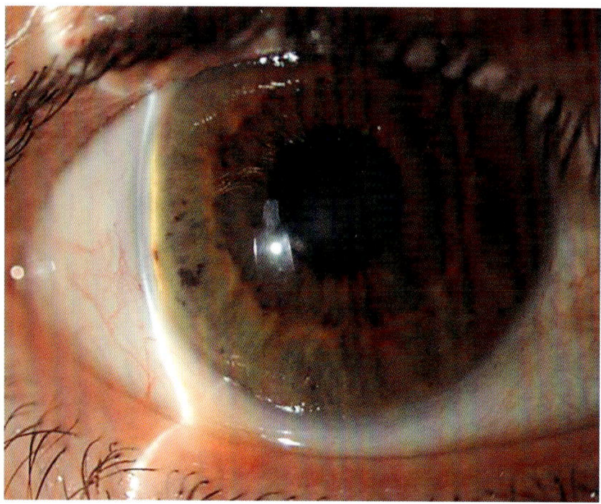

Fig. 2. The van Herick method. A very thin light beam is directed perpendicular to the surface of the eye at the limbus. In this case, the space between iris and corneal endothelium is <1/4 corneal thickness, suggesting a very narrow angle with possible ITC.

(grade 2, corresponding to an estimated angle of 20°), angle closure is considered possible, while grades 3 and 4 imply a low and very low risk of angle closure, respectively (fig. 2).

The van Herick method is very useful to identify the need for gonioscopy in patients not otherwise suspected of glaucoma, and narrower grades have been shown to be reliable indicators of the width of the angle on gonioscopy [22]. However, it cannot *substitute* gonioscopy, which remains the current reference method for assessing angle closure and is an essential part of all glaucoma patients [23].

Gonioscopy

Gonioscopy is used to determine the topography of the ACA, always taking into account the level of iris insertion (true or apparent), the shape of the peripheral iris profile, the width of the angle approach, the degree of trabecular pigmentation, and the presence of areas of iridotrabecular apposition or synechiae. Gonioscopy should be performed in a dark room, using the thinnest slit beam, taking care to avoid shining the light through the pupil in order to avoid pupil constriction.

The use of a grading system for gonioscopy is highly desirable because it allows the comparison of findings at different times and the classification of different patients, and stimulates the observer to use a systematic approach in evaluating angle anatomy. Several grading systems have been introduced, but the Spaeth Grading System is the only descriptive method including all the above parameters [1].

Angle width grading must be performed with the eye in primary position, and it is essential to instruct the patient to maintain the desired gaze direction. If the patient looks in the direction of the mirror, the angle appears wider and vice versa: this can be useful to improve the visualization of the angle recess in narrow angles but may lead to misclassifications at the same time. Similarly, inadvertent pressure on the cornea may give an erroneously wide appearance of the angle. However, if properly performed, this maneuver modifies the relative position of the angle structures, thus allowing a 'dynamic' assessment of the angle. The so-called *dynamic indentation gonioscopy* is extremely useful and probably essential for a correct classification and a therapeutic approach to angle closure.

During indentation, the pressure applied on the center of the cornea pushes the aqueous posteriorly, forcing the iris against the lens and creating a flap valve effect, which prevents aqueous from moving through the pupil into the posterior chamber and forces it into the angle recess [3]. In appositional angle closure, the angle can be reopened by this force, while if there are adhesions between the iris and the TM (i.e. goniosynechiae) the corresponding portion of the angle remains closed [1]. Although, with practice, the rim of a Goldmann lens can also be used to indent the central cornea [4], it is recommended to use a small-diameter (e.g. 4-mirror) lens to perform the procedure.

Dynamic indentation gonioscopy is then essential to differentiate optical from either appositional or synechial closure, and should be performed in all cases (fig. 3). It can give precious information

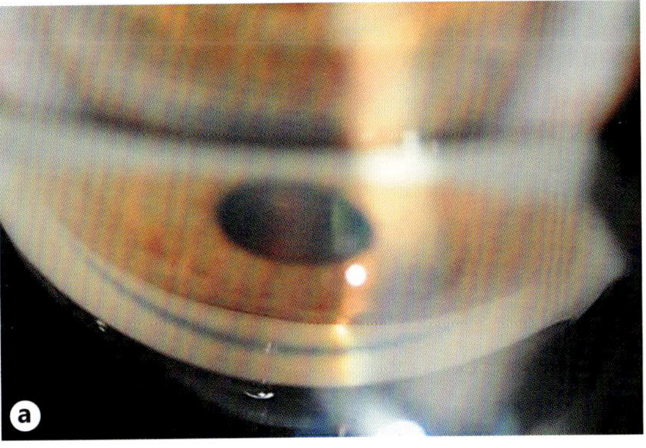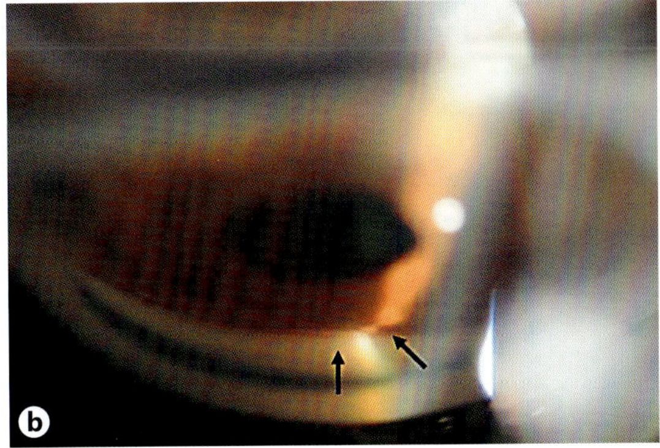

Fig. 3. Dynamic gonioscopy. **a** No structures visible in primary position. **b** During indentation (4-mirror lens), the TM becomes visible together with the sclera spur (left arrow); note the change in peripheral iris shape (right arrow). In this patient, indentation could induce only slight changes to the angle recess, suggesting that besides pupillary block, either a lens or a plateau iris-related mechanism could be involved.

also in more complex and less frequent situations, e.g. in plateau iris configuration. In pupillary block, the peripheral iris is held in its anterior position because of the little but relatively significant pressure gradient existing between the posterior and the anterior chamber. During indentation, the iris can easily move posteriorly because of the minimal resistance offered by the aqueous behind the iris plane to the force of indentation. In plateau iris configuration, the narrow angle appearance is due to a variation in ciliary body anatomy. During indentation, much more force than in pupillary block is needed to open the angle since the ciliary body must be displayed and the physical presence of the lens behind the iris plane tends to prevent posterior movement of the central iris. A sinuous configuration ('double hump') results, in which the iris follows the curvature of the lens, reaches its deepest point at the lens equator, then rises again over the ciliary processes before dropping peripherally. Similarly, an anteriorly positioned, enlarged, and/or intumescent lens, which physically pushes forward the iris plane, will offer high resistance to indentation: slight opening of the angle must be expected during gonioscopy when anomalies of the lens represent the predominant mechanism of angle closure [3].

Anterior Segment Imaging Techniques
In the last years, different AS imaging instruments have been commercialized and evolved mainly from research purposes to viable adjuncts to clinical examination. These are represented by ultrasound biomicroscopy (UBM), AS-OCT and Scheimpflug cameras. Added to gonioscopy, all can help elucidate the mechanism of angle closure in many cases. Interest towards alternative methods of angle assessment is encouraged by the need to supply the semiquantitative nature of gonioscopy and to reduce its substantial interobserver variability. Moreover, UBM has the potential to image simultaneously the ciliary body, posterior chamber, and the relationship between iris and lens [3], and is then very helpful in the diagnosis behind the iris (i.e. tumors or specific angle closure subtypes like plateau iris). Compared with UBM, AS-OCT achieves better resolution of ocular structures (about 18 µm for AS-OCT vs. about 50 µm for UBM) despite lower penetration, and is contact free [24]. Overall, image acquisition with AS-OCT is usually fast and easy, but results must be carefully analyzed in order to avoid misleading interpretation (fig. 4). The selection of a reference landmark for biometric analysis of the ACA is recommended with both AS-OCT and

UBM. All techniques do not rely on visible light and can be conducted in low-light or even dark conditions. Specifically, anterior segment OCT and Scheimpflug cameras are suitable for volumetric measurements and documentation of the dynamics of the chamber angle at different light conditions with the patient in the sitting position. Acquisitions can be performed also during corneal indentation, thus obtaining a real-time dynamic assessment of the angle which simulates dynamic indentation gonioscopy (fig. 5). Objective and quantitative angle assessment by imaging techniques have allowed to assess a range of new parameters, but currently they can provide information only on the examined sector and not about the whole circumference [25]. The new swept source OCT technology, with faster image acquisition, axial resolution of less than 10 μm and 360° scan protocols, seems to be promising in order to obtain a circumferential evaluation of the angle more similar to clinical gonioscopy.

At present, although the quantitative findings for both AS-OCT and UBM compare favorably to gonioscopy, none of the available imaging methods provide sufficient information about the anterior chamber anatomy to be considered a substitute for gonioscopy.

Treatment Options

Ideally, the aim of PACG treatment is to eliminate the underlying pathophysiological mechanism, thus reducing IOP. The choice of either the med-

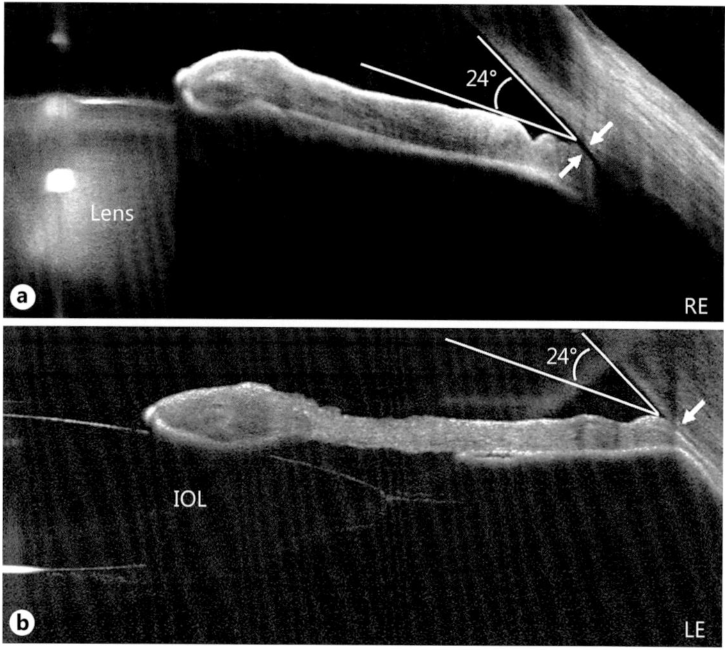

Fig. 4. AS-OCT imaging of the angle. The correct interpretation of the angle images requires careful observation. **a** A phakic eye with a 24° estimated angular width, but the correct angle recess is indicated by arrows and appears definitely narrower. The image shows some anomaly of the peripheral iris anatomy, suggesting a plateau iris conformation. **b** Fellow eye of the same patient. Phacoemulsification was performed after the detection of increased IOP and optic nerve head damage: the anterior chamber is significantly wider but the angle is closed (arrow). Phacoemulsification can prevent the formation of a synechial closure, but it cannot reverse it. RE = Right eye; LE = left eye.

Fig. 5. Dynamic OCT angle assessment. **a** The upper picture shows a very narrow angle imagined with an AS-OCT. The same angle is analyzed dynamically during corneal indentation performed with a scleral depressor (lower image): note the angle opening and the change in the iris shape induced by the indention. **b** The upper picture shows a closed angle; during indentation, the iris is pushed posteriorly by the force of indentation, but the angle recess does not open because of a synechial closure.

(For figure see next page.)

Bagnis · Traverso

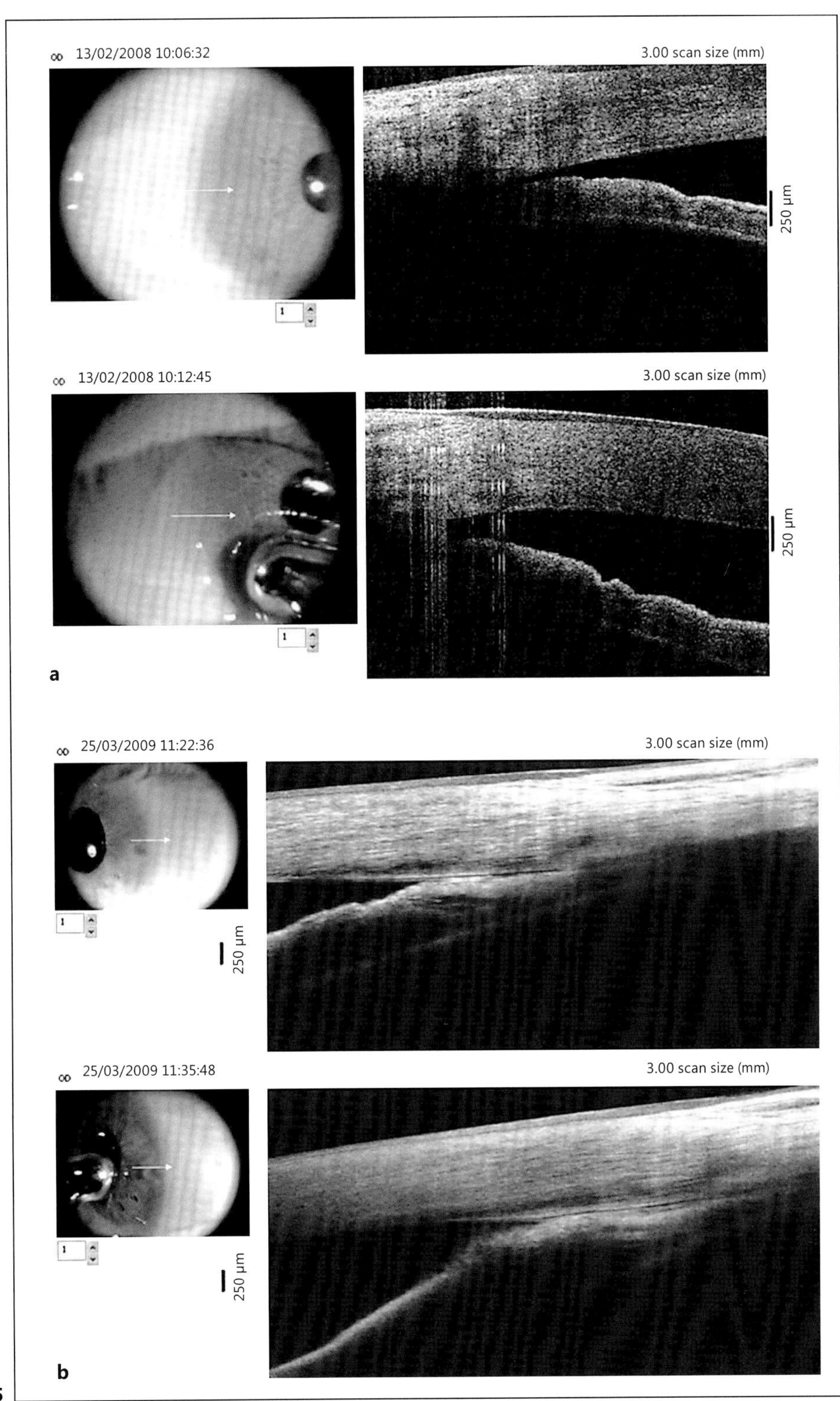

13/02/2008 10:06:32
3.00 scan size (mm)
250 µm
1
13/02/2008 10:12:45
3.00 scan size (mm)
250 µm
1
a
25/03/2009 11:22:36
3.00 scan size (mm)
250 µm
1
25/03/2009 11:35:48
3.00 scan size (mm)
250 µm
1
b
5

ical, laser, or surgical therapeutic approach must be based on an overall evaluation of each case.

General Rules

- Nd:YAG/argon laser peripheral iridotomy (LPI; seldom by surgical iridectomy) for pupillary block in order to eliminate the pressure gradient between the posterior and the anterior iris surface. It is recommendable to make sure that a patent iridotomy is present/made before considering mechanisms other than pupillary block (guidelines). Since complications of iridotomy are uncommon, its use as the initial procedure is justified practically in every case [1].
- Argon laser peripheral iridoplasty, for plateau iris in order to shrink the peripheral iris, contracting and flatting its peripheral curvature thus widening the angle approach and eliminating appositional closure. Iridotomy is anyway essential to confirm the diagnosis of plateau iris syndrome and should be performed first also in cases of supposed combined pupillary block and plateau iris configuration [26].
- Lens extraction when a phacomorphic component exists.
- Trabeculectomy is performed for the treatment of CACG whenever either medical and/or laser treatments are ineffective. The procedure can be also performed combined with cataract extraction.

Specific Treatment

AAC attack is an ophthalmologic emergency in which the priorities are:

- To break the attack and lower IOP
- To safeguard the fellow eye.

Medical treatment aims at lowering IOP and relieving symptoms and signs so that laser iridotomy is possible. Topical miotics (pilocarpine 2% or dapiprazole), a topical β-blocker, a topical α$_2$-agonist, and a topical steroid are given immediately along with an osmotic agent or acetazolamide. When the sphincter is ischemic (i.e. IOP >50 mm Hg), multiple applications of parasympathomimetics are not helpful, will not cause pupillary constriction, and may cause forward rotation of the ciliary muscle thus increasing the pupillary block.

LPI should be attempted if the cornea is sufficiently clear and a prophylactic one has always to be considered in the fellow eye. Laser iridotomy appears effective in preventing long-term IOP rises in around 90% of contralateral fellow eyes of those who have suffered an AAC [4]. On the contrary, it is not effective in reversing synechial angle closure. Argon laser iridotomy is rarely performed nowadays, but thermal laser pretreatment of dark and thick irides reduces the total YAG energy required. If the cornea is cloudy, a surgical iridectomy can be considered as an alternative to laser iridotomy. All the potential risks and benefits of this intraocular surgical procedure must be evaluated in each case individually.

Besides the specific indication for plateau iris syndrome, laser peripheral iridoplasty has been reported to be as or more effective than medical therapy to break an AAC, and it is currently used by some glaucoma specialists when topical treatment and oral acetazolamide are not effective within 1 h [27]. This technique is ineffective and probably detrimental in case of synechial angle closure.

Clear cornea peripheral paracentesis at the slit lamp under topical anesthesia can also be considered to immediately lower the IOP and instantaneously relieve symptoms preventing further damage to both the optic nerve head and the TM secondary to acute IOP increase [28, 29]. Besides the generous instillation of antiseptics before and after the procedure (e.g. povidone-iodine 5%), it is recommended to use a fine needle (e.g. 30 G) to make the corneal tract in order to obtain a significant but not excessively rapid IOP lowering and prevent choroidal effusions or hemorrhages.

According to the main mechanism determining angle occlusion, pupillary constriction, iridotomy, iridoplasty, or lens extraction should be considered in case of intermittent angle closure.

Medical treatment alone is rarely effective during CACG, and an iridotomy/iridectomy is al-

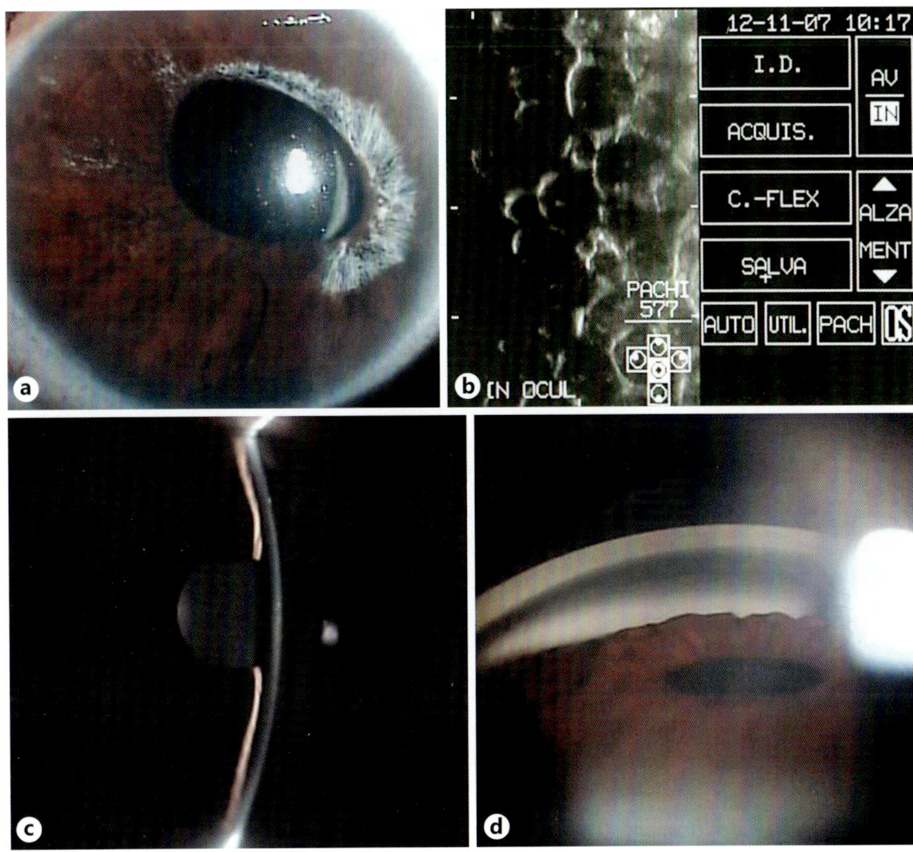

Fig. 6. a APAC eye after phacoemulsification and intraocular lens implant. Despite a prompt initial medical treatment and a successful LPI, the IOP did not normalize in this patient after an AAC attack. Early phacoemulsification was then performed. The BCVA is now 1.0 and the IOP 16 mm Hg with timolol 0.5% t.i.d. Note the iris torsion, a localized subatrophy and the irregular pupil. **b** Endothelial microscopy of the same eye. The endothelial cell count was dramatically reduced: both the APAC itself and the phacoemulsification may cause a significant endothelial cell loss in such cases. **c** Fellow eye of the same patient. Note the extremely shallow anterior chamber due to a thicker than normal lens. BCVA is presently 0.9. **d** Gonioscopic view of the same eye. In primary position, the angular recess is completely obscured by the iris profile despite a patent LPI and during dynamic gonioscopy (not shown in the picture) the angle widened minimally. The lens-related component is likely to play a pivotal role in this case. The lens-related component is likely in this eye.

ways required to relief any pupillary block. The latter may be sufficient to control IOP if the synechial closure is less than half the circumference, but topical adjunctive hypotensive medications are often required to reduce IOP during CACG [30] Laser trabeculoplasty is not indicated in these cases as it may increase synechial formation. Lens extraction should be considered possibly combined with a filtering procedure in case of uncontrolled IOP.

Any lens-related component involved in angle closure persists despite a patent LPI. Data concerning long-term IOP after acute PAC (APAC) show that a rise in IOP requiring treatment can occur in more than 50% of patients treated with LPI and up to 30% of those treated with laser peripheral iridoplasty plus LPI [31, 32]. Phacoemulsification with intraocular lens implantation has been proposed in the treatment of both CACG and AAC glaucoma. Concerning AAC, the aim of early phacoemulsification is to eliminate or at least reduce the risk of recurrent acute reclosure, the formation of PAS, and the development of CACG [33]. Any lens-related mechanism involved in the angle closure persists despite a patent LPI. Long-term data show that up to 20–25% of patients still have residual appositional angle closure despite a successful LPI and that a rise in IOP requiring treatment can occur in more than 50% of patients treated with LPI and up to 30% of those treated with laser peripheral iridoplasty plus LPI after APAC [31, 32, 34, 35]. The exact mechanisms through which cataract extraction effectively treats angle closure are not completely understood, but pupillary block relief and angle widening are likely to be the most important [33]. Indeed, phacoemulsification induces significant changes in the anterior chamber morphology, as demonstrated by imaging studies. After surgery, both the anterior chamber depth and volume increase, together with angle widening. Significant modifications in iris position and configuration also occur: in a phakic eye, the iris is attached to the lens and pushed forward, while it is shifted back and tends to remain free from an intraocular lens after phacoemulsification. Worthy of note, a postoperative increase in anterior chamber depth is not necessarily the same as *reopening* of a closed angle or *PAS resolution* (fig. 4). The extent and the degree of PAS can influence IOP control in both AAC and CACG; whether phacoemulsification will be effective in lowering IOP depends essentially on the irreversible damage to the TM during angle closure. A recent iris apposition with subsequent severe IOP increase may have a better prognosis than a long-standing synechial closure with even lower IOP values [36].

Clear lens extraction has also been proposed as a treatment option, and one prospective multicenter clinical trial has recently adressed this issue [37–39].

However, despite several data in support of phacoemulsification with intraocular lens implantation as a safe and effective procedure for both APAC and CACG, the appropriate role for lens extraction in the management of the disease is still to be defined. As a general rule, cataract removal may be considered at all stages in case of CACG since it can effectively eradicate angle closure and allow sufficient IOP control [1]. Clear lens extraction should be considered only if the angle does not open with a patent LPI and IOP is not properly controlled in the presence of unquestionable glaucomatous damage [1]. It is plausible that clear lens extraction provides the same benefits as a visually significant cataract extraction, but the risk:benefit ratio would probably be greater.

The risk of both intraoperative and postoperative complications in angle closure is higher than in normal eyes because of the shallow anterior chamber, larger lens, corneal edema, poorly dilated or miotic pupil, lower endothelial cell count, and weaker zonulas especially after an AAC attack (fig. 6) [6]. Necessary precautions (i.e. preoperative intravenous mannitol or adjunctive viscoelastic use) must be taken into account when considering surgery in such cases and any potential benefit of an incisional procedure should be weighed against the risk of intervention.

References

1 Classification and terminology – primary angle closure; in European Glaucoma Society: Terminology and Guidelines for Glaucoma, ed 4. Savona, PubliComm, 2014, pp 100–113.

2 Traverso CE, Bagnis A, Bricola G: Angle-closure glaucoma; in Yanoff M, Duker JS (eds): Ophthalmology, ed 2. St. Louis, Mosby, 2004, pp 1491–1498.

3 Teng CC, Liebmann JM, Tello C, Ritch R, Greenfiled DS: Angle closure glaucomas; in Choplin NT, Traverso CE (eds): Atlas of Glaucoma, ed 3. Boca Raton, Taylor & Francis, 2014, pp 127–163.

4 Foster P, Low S: Primary angle-closure glaucoma; in Shaarawy TM, Sherwood MB, Hitchings RA, Crowston JG (eds): Glaucoma – Medical Diagnosis & Therapy (vol 1). Philadelphia, Saunders Elsevier, 2009, pp 327–337.

5 Sihota R, Lakshimaiah NC, Walia KB, et al: The trabecular meshwork in acute and chronic angle closure glaucoma. Indian J Ophthalmol 2001;49:255–249.

6 Day AC, Baio G, Gazzard G, et al: The prevalence of primary angle closure glaucoma in European derived populations: a systematic review. Br J Ophthalmol 2012;96:1162–1167.

7 Ng WS, Ang GS, Azuara-Blanco A: Primary angle closure glaucoma: a descriptive study in Scottish Caucasians. Clin Experiment Ophthalmol 2008;36:847–845.

8 He M, Foster PJ, Johnson GJ, Khaw PT: Angle-closure glaucoma in East Asian and European people. Different diseases (review)? Eye 2006;20:3–12.

9 Ang LP, Ang LP: Current understanding of the treatment and outcome of acute primary angle-closure glaucoma: an Asian perspective. Ann Acad Med Singapore 2008;37:210–215.

10 Friedman DS, Gazzard G, Min CB, et al: Age and sex variation in angle findings among normal Chinese subjects: a comparison of UBM, Scheimpflug and gonioscopic assessment of the anterior chamber angle. J Glaucoma 2008;17:5–10.

11 Alsbirk PH: Anatomical risk factors in primary angle-closure glaucoma. A ten year follow-up survey based on limbal and axial anterior chamber depths in a high risk population. Int Ophthalmol 1992;16:265–272.

12 Tun TI, Baskaran M, Perera SA, et al: Sectorial variations of iridocorneal angle width and iris volume in Chinese Singaporeans: a swept-source optical coherence tomography study. Graefes Arch Clin Exp Ophthalmol 2014;252:1127–1132.

13 Quigley HA, Silver DM, Friedman DS, et al: Iris cross-sectional area decreases with pupil dilation and its dynamic behavior is a risk factor in angle closure. J Glaucoma 2009;18:173–179.

14 Quigley HA: The iris is a sponge: a cause of angle closure. Ophthalmology 2010; 117:1–2.

15 Chakravarti T, Spaeth GL: The prevalence of myopia in eyes with angle closure. J Glaucoma 2007;16:642–643.

16 Chong GT, Wen JC, Su DH, et al: Ocular biometrics of myopic eyes with narrow angles. J Glaucoma 2016;25:140–144.

17 Keenan TD, Salmon JF, Yeates D, et al: Trends in rates of primary angle closure glaucoma and cataract surgery in England from 1968 to 2004. J Glaucoma 2009;18:201–205.

18 Day AC, Foster PJ: Increases in rates of both laser peripheral iridotomy and phacoemulsification have accompanied a fall in acute angle closure rates in the UK. Br J Ophthalmol 2011;95:1339–1340.

19 Boland MV, Zhang L, Broman AT, et al: Comparison of optic nerve head topography and visual field in eyes with open-angle and angle-closure glaucoma. Ophthalmology 2008;115:239–245.

20 Bonomi L, Marraffa M, Marchini G, Canali N: Perimetric defects after a single acute angle-closure glaucoma attack. Graefes Arch Clin Exp Ophthalmol 1999;237:908–914.

21 Caprioli J, Sears M, Miller JM: Patterns of early visual field loss in open-angle glaucoma. Am J Ophthalmol 1987;103: 512–517.

22 Foster PJ, Devereux JG, Alsbirk PH, et al: Detection of gonioscopically occludable angles and primary angle closure glaucoma by estimation of limbal chamber depth in Asians: modified grading scheme. Br J Ophthalmol 2000;84:186–192.

23 Dabasia PL, Edgar DF, Murdoch IE, Lawrenson JG: Noncontact screening methods for the detection of narrow anterior chamber angles. Invest Ophthalmol Vis Sci 2015;6:3929–3935.

24 Seager FE, Wang J, Arora KS, Quigley HA: The effect of sclera spur identification methods on structural measurements by anterior segment optical coherence tomography. J Glaucoma 2014; 23:29–38.

25 Tun TA, Baskaran M, Prera SA, et al: Sectorial variations of iridocorneal angle width and iris volume in Chinese Singaporeans: a swept-source optical coherence tomography study. Graefes Arch Clin Exp Ophthalmol 2014;252:1127–1132.

26 Ritch R, Tham CC, Lam DS: Argon laser peripheral iridoplasty (ALPI): an update. Surv Ophthalmol 2007;52:279–288.

27 Lai JS, Tham CC, Chua JK, et al: To compare argon laser peripheral iridoplasty (ALPI) against systemic medications in treatment of acute primary angle-closure: mid-term results. Eye (Lond) 2006; 20:309–314.

28 Arnavielle S, Creuzot-Garcher C, Bron AM: Anterior chamber paracentesis in patients with acute elevation of intraocular pressure. Graefes Arch Clin Exp Ophthalmol 2007;245:345–350.

29 Lam JS, Chua JK, Tham CC, Lai JS: Efficacy and safety of immediate anterior chamber paracentesis in the treatment of acute primary angle-closure glaucoma: a pilot study. Ophthalmology 2002; 109:64–70.

30 Aung T, Chan YH, Chew PT; EXACT Study Group: Degree of angle closure and the intraocular pressure-lowering effect of latanoprost in subjects with chronic angle-closure glaucoma. Ophthalmology 2005;112:267–271.

31 Aung T, Ang LP, Chan SP, Chew PT: Acute primary angle-closure: long-term intraocular pressure outcome in Asian eyes. Am J Opthalmol 2001;131:7–12.

32 Lai JS, Tham CC, Chua JK, et al: Laser peripheral iridoplasty as initial treatment of acute attack of primary angle closure: a long-term follow-up study. J Glaucoma 2001;11:484–487.

33 Lam DS, Tham CC, Lai JS, Leung DY: Current approaches to the management of acute primary angle closure. Curr Opin Ophthalmol 2007;18:146–151.

34 He MG, Friedman DS, Ge J, et al: Laser peripheral iridotomy in primary angle-closure suspects: biometric and gonioscopic outcomes: the Liwan Eye Study. Ophthalmology 2007;114:494.

35 Gazzrd G, Friedman DS, Devereux JG, et al: A prospective ultrasound biomicroscopy evaluation in Asian eyes. Ophthalmology 2003;110:630–638.

36 Zhou YH, Wang M, Li Y, et al: Phacoemulsification treatment of subjects with acute primary angle closure and chronic primary angle-closure glaucoma. J Glaucoma 2009;18:464–451.

37 Thomas R, Walland MJ, Parikh RS: Clear lens extraction in angle closure glaucoma. Curr Opin Ophthalmol 2011; 22:110–114.

38 Azuara-Blanco A, Burr JM, Cochran C, et al: The effectiveness of early lens extraction with intraocular lens implantation for the treatment of primary angle-closure glaucoma (EAGLE): study protocol for a randomized controlled trial. Trials 2011;12:133.

39 Azuara-Blanco A, Burr J, Ramsay C, et al: The effectiveness of early lens extraction for the treatment of primary angle-closure glaucoma: a randomized controlled trial (EAGLE). Lancet 2016, in press.

Alessandro Bagnis, MD, PhD
Clinica Oculistica, Di.N.O.G.M.I. University of Genoa and
IRCCS Azienda Ospedaliera Universitaria San Martino IST
Viale Benedetto XV 7, IT–16132 Genoa (Italy)
E-Mail alebagnis@libero.it

Traverso CE, Stalmans I, Topouzis F, Bagnasco L (eds): Glaucoma.
ESASO Course Series. Basel, Karger, 2016, vol 8, pp 52–75 (DOI: 10.1159/000446142)

Treatment of Glaucoma with or without Medications Lowering Intraocular Pressure: Options and Relevant General Health Issues

John Thygesen

Department of Ophthalmology, Rigshospitalet, Copenhagen University Hospital, Glostrup, Denmark

Abstract

The etiology of glaucoma is multifactorial. Intraocular pressure (IOP) is the only modifiable factor in glaucoma management proven to alter the natural course of the disease. Currently, based on evidence-based glaucoma therapy, the only approach proven to be efficient in preserving visual function is lowering IOP. Lowering IOP by 20–40% has been shown to reduce the rate of progressive visual field loss by half. Despite the fact that IOP-lowering interventions reduce the risk of progression and delay the onset of glaucoma, its pathogenesis is controversial and not completely understood. In this matter, non-IOP-dependent risk factors appear to be responsible for around 50% of glaucoma cases. New drugs are now entering the clinic, along with new ways to deliver them. There is growing consensus that the future of glaucoma management will be based more on the optic nerve pathway from the retina to the visual cortex and will not be strictly limited to improving outflow or reducing inflow. But still, many future IOP-lowering options will be developed, including neuroprotective strategies aiming to directly prevent or significantly hinder neuronal cell damage. The goal of glaucoma treatment is to maintain the patient's visual function and related quality of life at a sustainable cost. The cost of treatment in terms of inconvenience and side effects as well as financial implications for the individual and society requires careful evaluation. In conclusion, IOP lowering is the only proven therapy for glaucoma at present. Neuroprotection may be clinically useful (based on one trial), but this needs to be confirmed. So far, we have no evidence of potential therapies related to ocular blood flow and glaucoma care, and evidence to support the use of acupuncture, vitamins, minerals, or herbal medicines such as marijuana for treating glaucoma is insufficient.

Introduction

The first part of the chapter is based upon the European Glaucoma Society (EGS) Guidelines 2014 (www.eugs.org).

Glaucoma refers to a group of eye conditions that cause chronic, progressive optic neuropathies with common morphological changes at the optic nerve head (ONH) and the retinal nerve fiber layer. These changes are associated with progressive retinal ganglion cell (RGC) death that may lead to characteristic damage to the visual field.

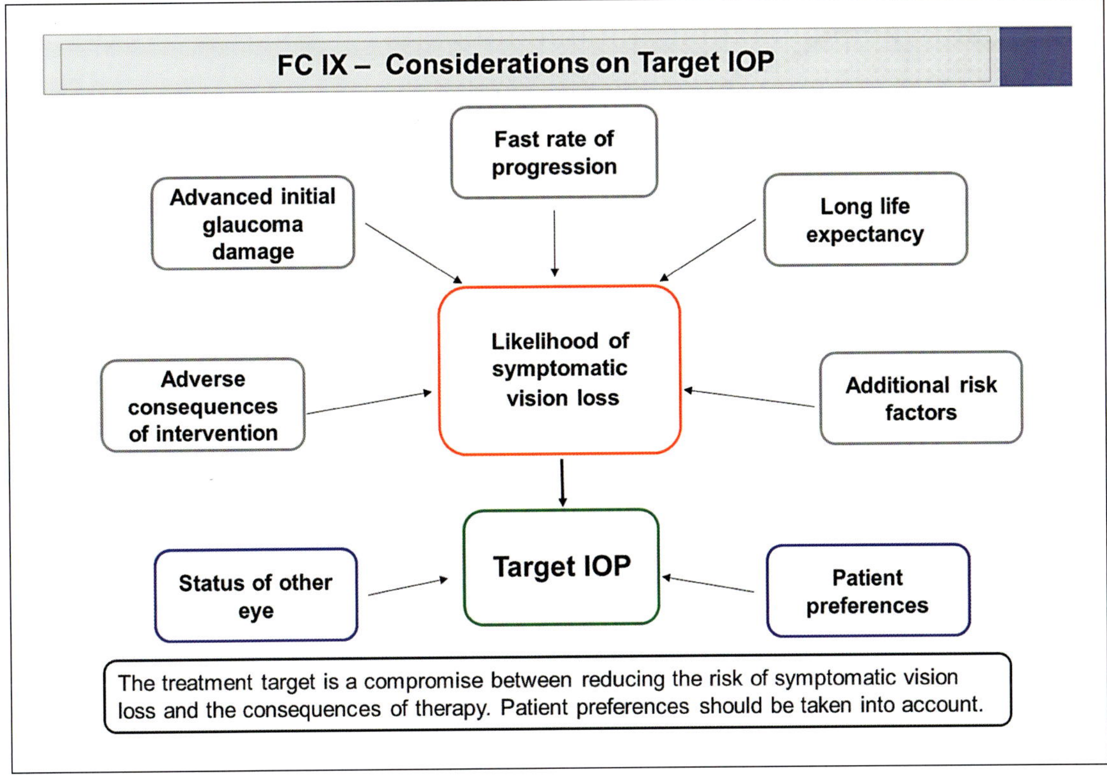

Fig. 1. Considerations on target IOP. Reprinted with permission from the European Glaucoma Society (EGS Guidelines 2014).

The most common subtype of glaucoma is primary open-angle glaucoma (POAG). Despite the normal clinical appearance of the drainage pathway, the aqueous outflow is restricted in most POAG cases. The increased intraocular pressure (IOP) that may follow is referred to as the main risk factor for glaucoma progression.

Glaucoma Therapy

Lowering Intraocular Pressure
Evidence-Based Glaucoma Therapy: Still to Lower Intraocular Pressure
The etiology of glaucoma is multifactorial. IOP is the only modifiable factor in glaucoma management proven to alter the natural course of the disease. Lowering IOP by 20–40% has been shown to reduce the rate of progressive visual field loss by half [1, 2]. Currently, the only approach proven to be efficient in preserving visual function is lowering IOP [3–5].

Despite the fact that IOP-lowering interventions reduce the risk of progression and delay the disease onset of glaucoma, its pathogenesis is controversial and not completely understood. In this matter, non-IOP-dependent risk factors appear to be responsible for around 50% of glaucoma cases [6].

Perfusion Pressure
Other possible treatment areas have been investigated, including ocular blood flow and neuroprotection. There are experimental as well popula-

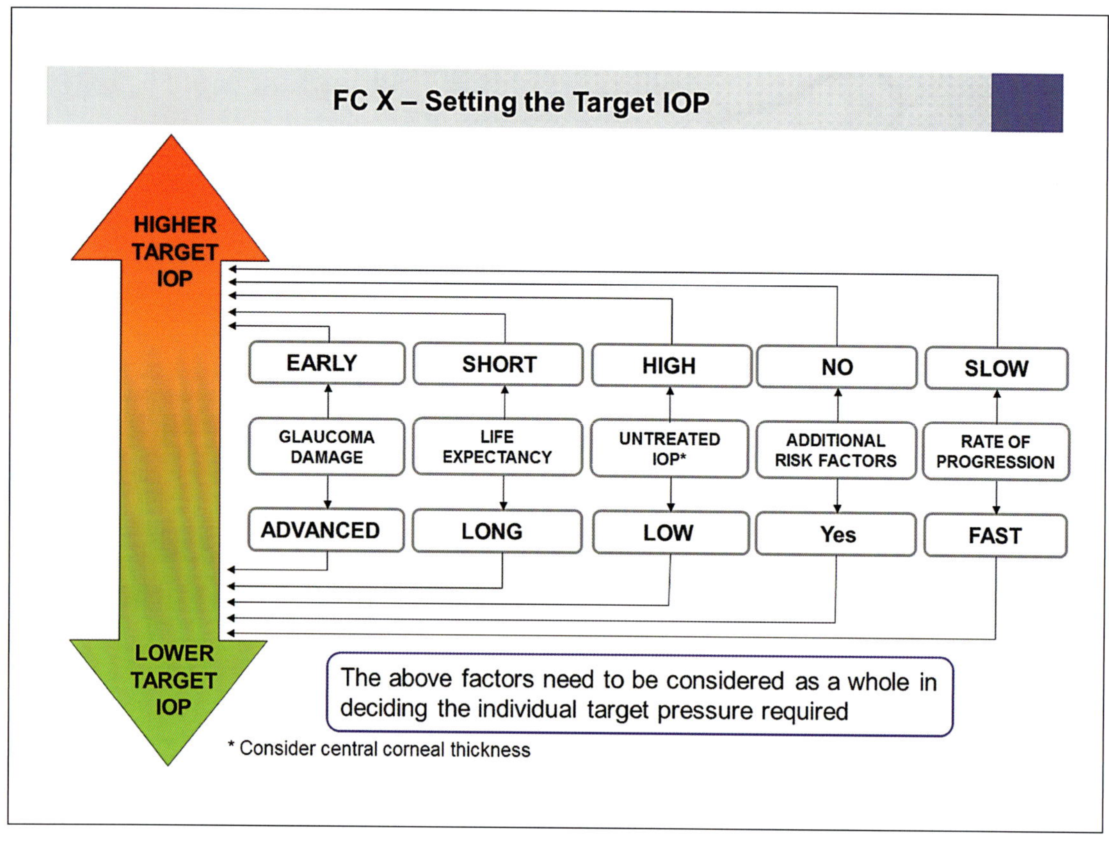

Fig. 2. Setting the target IOP. Reprinted with permission from the European Glaucoma Society (EGS Guidelines 2014).

tion-based studies indicating that perfusion pressure may be relevant in glaucoma [7–10] but very difficult to measure. An increase in IOP will lead to a reduction in perfusion pressure. Blood pressure levels may also be important in glaucoma. However, there is no conclusive evidence to support the idea that perfusion pressure can be increased by manipulating blood pressure or ocular blood flow in glaucoma patients.

Neuroprotection

Neuroprotection can be defined as a 'therapeutic approach' aiming to directly prevent, hinder, and, in some cases, reverse neuronal cell damage. Since glaucoma can continue deteriorating in spite of an apparently well-controlled IOP, the need for effective non-IOP-related treatments is widely acknowledged. Several compounds have been shown to be neuroprotective in animal models of experimental glaucoma. So far, no compound has reached a sufficient level of evidence to be considered as a neuroprotectant in humans. A large long-term randomized trial using a neuroprotective agent, memantine, was analyzed several years ago, but with negative results. A more recent study claiming that topical brimonidine might have neuroprotective properties in glaucoma patients has been questioned in a systematic review on neuroprotection in glaucoma [11, 12].

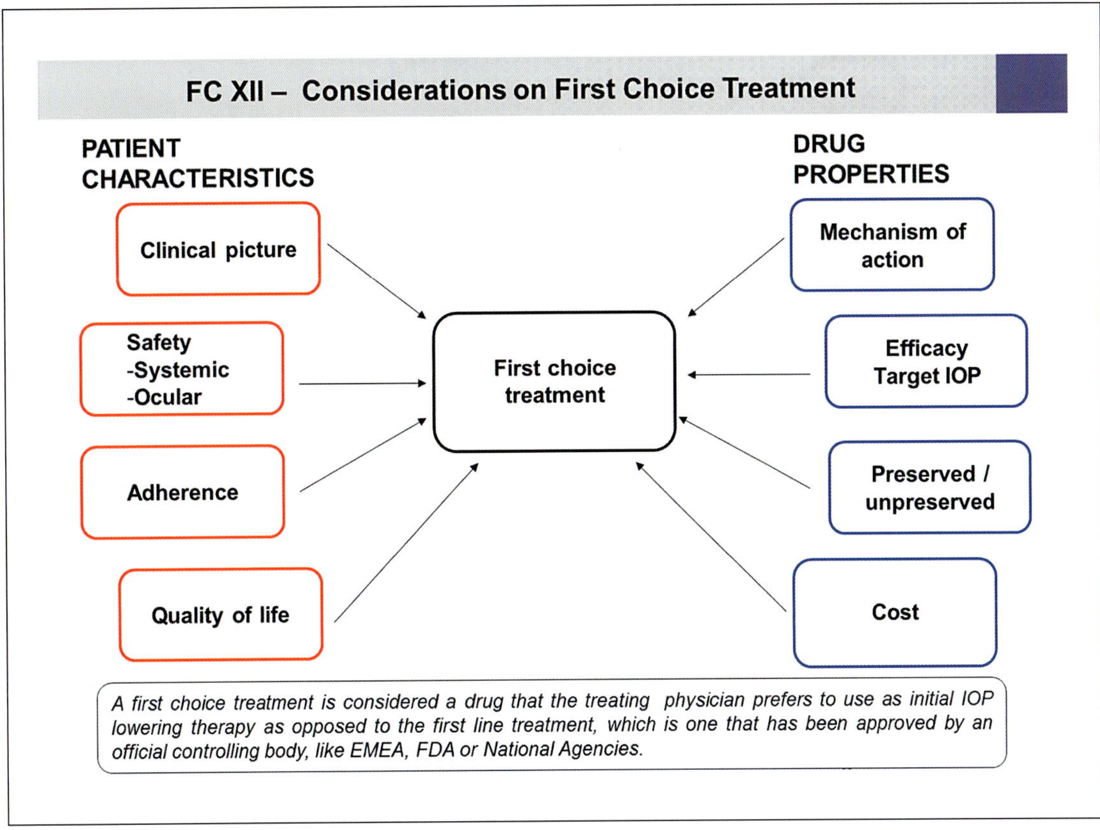

Fig. 3. Considerations on first-choice treatment. Reprinted with permission from the European Glaucoma Society (EGS Guidelines 2014).

Target Intraocular Pressure

Therapy in glaucoma management aims to lower IOP to slow the rate of visual field deterioration.

Target IOP is the upper limit of the IOP estimated to be compatible with a rate of progression sufficiently slow to maintain vision-related quality of life in the expected lifetime of the patient. It should be reevaluated regularly and, additionally, when progression of disease is identified or when ocular or systemic comorbidities develop.

There is no single target IOP level that is appropriate for every patient, so the target IOP needs to be estimated separately for each eye of every patient (fig. 1–3).

Antiglaucoma Drugs

Several prospective randomized multicenter controlled clinical studies have clearly established the benefits of IOP reduction in managing POAG at various stages of the disease whether of the 'high-pressure' or 'normal-pressure' variety as well as reducing the conversion of ocular hypertension to POAG [13–17].

Most forms of open-angle glaucoma and many types of chronic angle closure glaucoma are initially treated with topical and occasionally orally administrated agents that act either on the reduction of aqueous humor production or enhancement of the aqueous outflow, or on both. Although acute

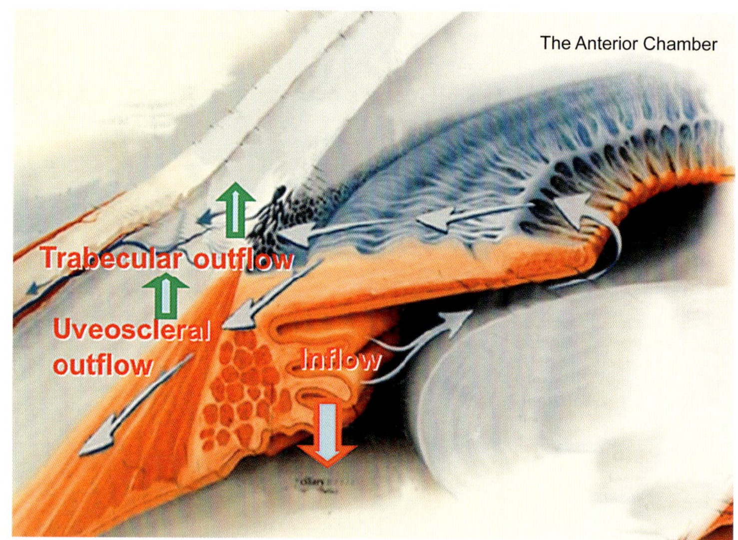

Fig. 4. Mechanisms of IOP-lowering medications.

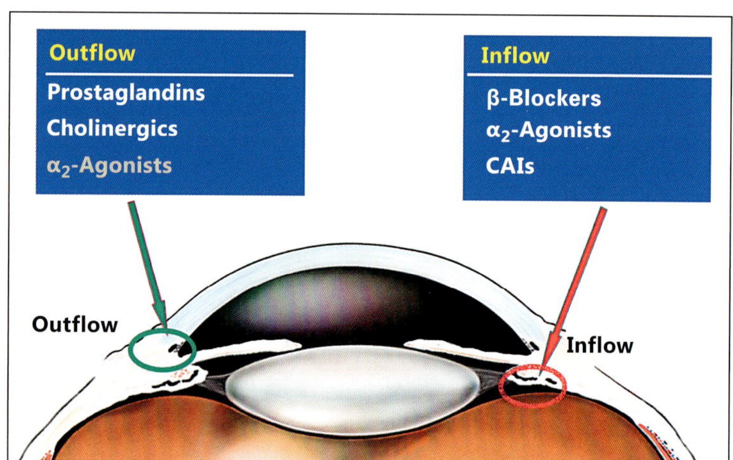

Fig. 5. Mechanisms of IOP-lowering medications for glaucoma treatment.

angle closure with or without glaucoma needs rapid laser or incisional surgery, medical treatment will usually be initiated as a first step in most cases.

Laser treatment may be a suitable first option for patients with known intolerance or allergy to topical agents, or suspected poor compliance.

When initially selecting medical therapy it is important to consider some relevant patient characteristics as well as features related to the drug.

Current glaucoma treatment is directed at *lowering IOP*. Future strategies of glaucoma treatment aim at *neuroprotection, neuroregulation* and *improved optic nerve perfusion*.

Mechanisms of Glaucoma Medications: Current Treatment

An Overview of Currently Available Intraocular Pressure-Lowering Glaucoma Medications
Overall, the current available glaucoma eye drops all seek to decrease IOP. They can be grouped into therapeutic agents that decrease the production

IOP lowering effect of glaucoma drugs:
meta-analysis of randomised controlled trials

Generic name	Difference from baseline %	
	Peak %	*Trough %*
Bimatoprost	-33	-28
Travoprost	-31	-29
Latanoprost	-31	-28
Timolol	-27	-26
Brimonidine	-25	-18
Betaxolol	-23	-20
Dorzolamide (x2 or 3)	-22	-17
Brinzolamide (x3)	-17	-17

Fig. 6. Effect of IOP-lowering glaucoma drugs: a meta-analysis of randomized controlled trials reported by van der Valk et al. [18]. Reprinted with permission from John Thygesen.

of aqueous humor production and/or increase the drainage through the trabecular meshwork (TM), and/or increase uveoscleral outflow (fig. 4, 5). The various drugs differ in their effectiveness, side effect profile, dosing schedule, and costs.

Currently, the following medical IOP-lowering treatments are available for glaucoma.

Prostaglandin analogs: tafluprost, latanoprost, bimatoprost, travoprost, and unoprostone isopropyl.

β-Blockers: timolol, levobunolol, carteolol, metipranolol, betatoxol, and nipradilol.

Carbonic anhydrase inhibitors (CAIs): dorzolamide, brinzolamide, acetazolamide (topical and oral medication), and methazolamide (oral medication).

Sympathomimetic drugs: α_2-selective adrenergic receptor agonists brimonidine and apracloni-dine, and α- and β-adrenergic agonists (α and β receptors) epinephrine/adrenalin and dipivefrin.

Parasympathomimetic drugs (cholinergics): pilocarpine and echothiophate.

Hypertonic or osmotic agents: glycerol (oral), mannitol (intravenous), and isosorbide.

Prostaglandin Analogs
Prostaglandins are the most potent IOP-lowering drugs, lowering the IOP by 28–33 mm Hg at peak. The primary mechanism of action of prostaglandins is to increase uveoscleral outflow, reducing IOP by 25–35% (fig. 6). Reduction in IOP starts approximately 2–4 h after the first administration, with the peak effect within approximately 8–12 h. Thus, IOP measurements taken in the morning represent the peak effect of prostaglandin analogs taken in the evening.

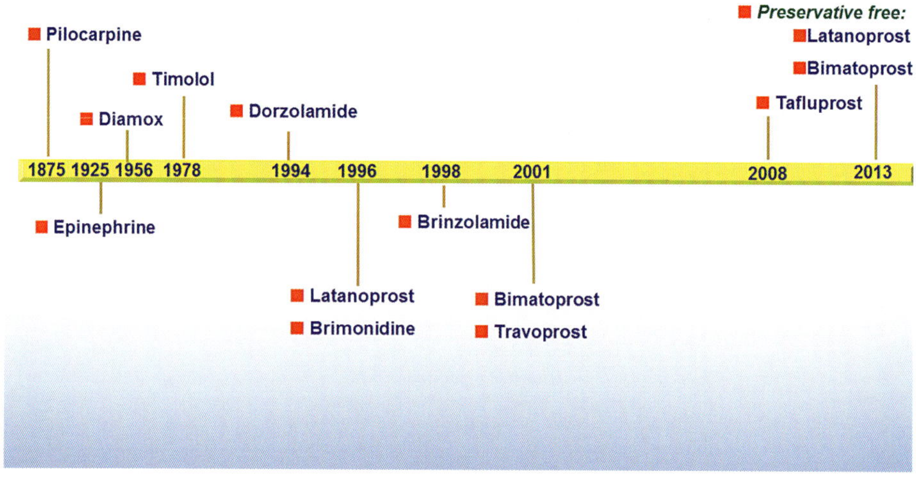

Fig. 7. Topical IOP-lowering monotherapy available from 1875 to 2015. Reprinted with permission from John Thygesen.

Clinical trials that measured 24-hour IOP suggested that evening administration is generally preferable because it gave a better circadian IOP profile.

Maximum IOP lowering is often achieved 3–5 weeks from commencement of treatment. Differences among drugs within this class in the capability of reducing IOP did not exceed 1 mm Hg.

The most common adverse effects are conjunctival hyperemia or irritation, a change in eye color (mostly in hazel or green eyes), and an increase in thickness and length of eyelashes. Prostaglandin analogs may also cause periocular skin pigmentation, iritis, and cystoid macular edema. Latanoprost requires refrigeration.

In addition, prostaglandin administration has been reported to result in recurrence of corneal epithelium herpes and should therefore be used with caution in these patients.

No significant systemic adverse reactions have been associated with the use of prostaglandins. Today, prostaglandins are the most frequently used first-line and first-choice antiglaucoma medications, and they are available in many different generic options. Since their development in the 1990s, prostaglandin derivatives (latanoprost, travoprost, bimatoprost, and tafluprost) (fig. 7, 8) have progressively replaced β-blockers as first-choice/first-line therapy. This is mainly because they are the most effective IOP-lowering agents (fig. 6) [18], lack relevant systemic side effects, and require just once-daily administration. Recently, a number of latanoprost generics as well as preservative-free and benzalkonium chloride (BAK)-free prostaglandin formulations have entered the glaucoma market.

Details on the mode of action, IOP-lowering effect, contraindications, and side effects of other

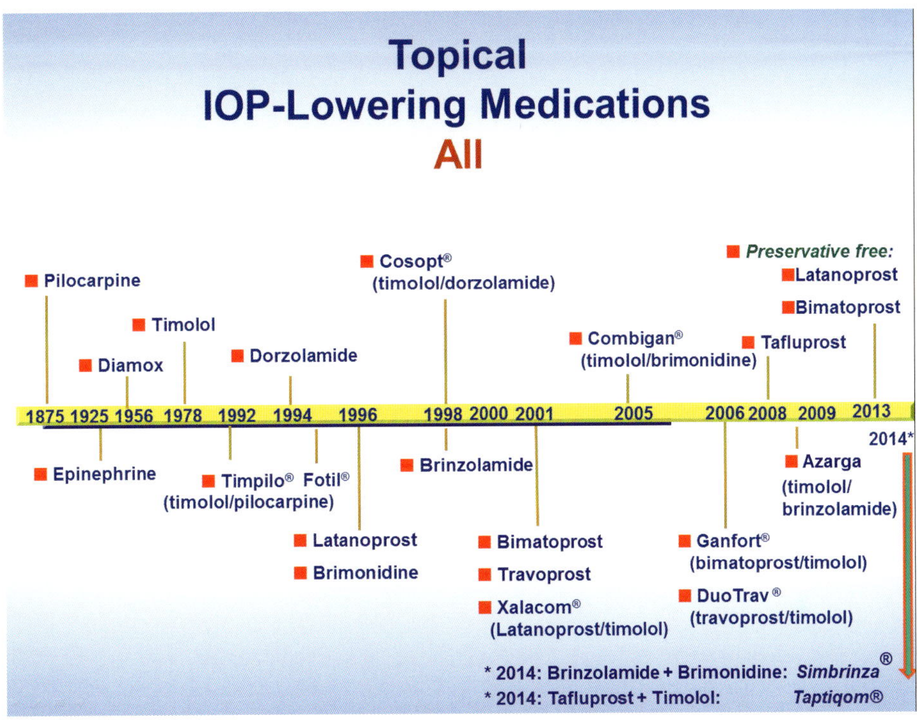

Fig. 8. All topical IOP-lowering mono- or combination therapies available from 1875 to 2015. Reprinted with permission from John Thygesen.

Table 1. Prostaglandin analogs

Compound	Mode of action	IOP reduction	Contraindications

Prostaglandin analogs
   Latanoprost 0.005%
   Tafluprost 0.0015%
   Travoprost 0.003–0.004%
Prostamides
   Bimatoprost 0.03%
   Bimatoprost 0.01%
	Increases uveoscleral outflow	25–35%	Contact lenses (unless reinserted 15 min following administration of the drugs)

Local side effects Conjunctival hyperemia, burning, stinging, foreign body sensation, itching, increased pigmentation of periocular skin, periorbital fat atrophy, eyelash changes, increased iris pigmentation (in green-brown, blue/gray-brown, or yellow-brown irides), cystoid macular edema (aphakic/pseudophakic patients) with posterior lens capsule rupture, or in eyes with known risk factors for macular edema, reactivation of herpes keratitis, uveitis			
Systemic side effects Dyspnea, chest pain/angina, muscle-back pain, exacerbation of asthma			

Table 2. β-Blockers or β-receptor antagonists

Compound	Mode of action	IOP reduction	Contraindications
Nonselective compound Timolol 0.1/0.25/0.5% Levobunolol 0.25% Metipranolol 0.1–0.3% Carteolol 0.5–2% Befunolol 0.5%	Decreases aqueous humor production	20–25%	Asthma, history of chronic obstructive pulmonary disease, sinus bradycardia (<60 beats/min), heart block, cardiac failure

Local side effects
    Conjunctiva hyperemia, superficial punctate keratitis, dry eye, corneal anesthesia, allergic blepharoconjunctivitis
Systemic side effects
    Bradycardia, arrhythmia, heart failure, syncope, bronchospasm, airway obstruction, distal edema, hypotension
    Hypoglycemia may be masked in insulin-dependent diabetes mellitus
    Nocturnal systemic hypotension, depression, sexual dysfunction			

β_1-*Selective compound* Betaxolol 0.5%	Decreases aqueous humor production	±20%	Asthma, history of chronic obstructive pulmonary disease, sinus bradycardia (<60 beats/min), heart block, cardiac-coronary failure

Local side effects
    Burning, stinging more pronounced than with nonselective compounds
Systemic side effects
    Respiratory and cardiac side effects less pronounced than with nonselective compounds
    Depression, erectile dysfunction			

Table 3. Carbonic anhydrase inhibitors

Compound	Mode of action	IOP reduction	Contraindications
Topical compound Brinzolamide 1% Dorzolamide 2%	Decreases aqueous humor production	20%	Patients with low corneal endothelial cell count due to increased risk of corneal edema

Local side effects
    Burning, stinging, bitter taste, superficial punctate keratitis, blurred vision, tearing
Systemic side effects
    Headache, urticaria, angioedema, pruritus, asthenia, dizziness, paresthesia, transient myopia			

Systemic compound Acetazolamide Methazolamide Dichlorphenamide	Decreases aqueous humor production	30–40%	Depressed sodium and/or potassium blood levels, cases of kidney and liver disease or dysfunction, suprarenal gland failure, hyperchloremic acidosis

Systemic side effects
    Paresthesia, hearing dysfunction, tinnitus, loss of appetite, taste alteration, nausea, vomiting, diarrhea,
    depression, decreased libido, kidney stones, blood dyscrasias, metabolic acidosis, electrolyte imbalance			

Table 4. α_2-Selective adrenergic agonists

Compound	Mode of action	IOP reduction	Contraindications
Apraclonidine 0.5–1.0%	Decreases aqueous humor production	25–35%	
Brimonidine 0.2%	Decreases aqueous humor production and increases uveoscleral outflow	18–25%	Oral monoamine oxidase inhibitor users Pediatric age Very low body weight in adults
Clonidine 0.125–0.5%	Decrease aqueous humor production	18–25%	

Local side effects
    Lid retraction, conjunctival blanching, limited mydriasis (apraclonidine), allergic blepharoconjunctivitis, periocular contact dermatitis, allergy or delayed hypersensitivity (apraclonidine and clonidine > brimonidine)
Systemic side effects
    Dry mouth and nose (apraclonidine), systemic hypotension, bradycardia (clonidine), fatigue, sleepiness (brimonidine)

Table 5. Nonselective adrenergics

Compound	Mode of action	IOP reduction	Contraindications
Epinephrine 0.25–2.0% Dipivefrin 0.1%	Decreases aqueous humor production and may increase uveoscleral outflow	15–20%	Occludable angles (iridotomy needed) Aphakic patients (macular edema)

Local side effects
    Conjunctival hyperemia and pigmentation, burning, stinging, ocular pain, blurred vision, macular edema
Systemic side effects
    Systemic hypertension, headache, anxiety, confusion, chest pain, shortness of breath, tachycardia, sweating

first-line drugs (β-blockers, CAIs, and α_2-selective adrenergic agonists) and second-line drugs are listed in tables 1–7.

β-Blockers (β-Receptor Antagonists)

β-Blockers reduce the production of aqueous humor by blocking β-receptors in the ciliary body. They have been used since 1978 (fig. 7). Nonselective β-blockers lower IOP by 4–6 mm Hg (20–25%), and the selective β_1-blocker betaxolol lowers it by 3–4 mm Hg (15–25%) (fig. 6). All β-blockers are less effective in eyes with dark irides.

Ocular adverse reactions include conjunctival allergies, conjunctival injection, and corneal epithelium disorders. Corneal sensitivity may be reduced. One major challenge for the use of β-blockers is their frequent systemic adverse effects due to their activation of both β_1- and β_2-receptors. In this matter, adverse effects of the respiratory system by β_2-blockers include worsening of asthma attacks and chronic obstructive pulmonary disease.

The most critical adverse effects of β_1-blockage are reduced heart rate and reduced cardiac contractility. Hence, β-blockers should be used with

Table 6. Parasympathomimetics (cholinergic drugs or miotics)

Compound	Mode of action	IOP reduction	Contraindications
Direct-acting compound Pilocarpine 0.5–4% Carbachol 0.75–3%	Facilitates aqueous outflow by contraction of the ciliary muscle, tension on the scleral spur and traction on TM	20–25%	Postoperative inflammation, uveitis neovascular glaucoma, risk of retinal detachment, spastic gastrointestinal disturbances, peptic ulcer, pronounced bradycardia, hypotension, recent myocardial infarction, epilepsy, parkinsonism

Local side effects
    Reduced vision due to miosis and accommodative myopia, conjunctival hyperemia, retinal detachment, lens opacities, precipitation of angle closure, iris cysts
Systemic side effects
    Intestinal cramps, bronchospasm, headache

Compound	Mode of action	IOP reduction	Contraindications
Indirect-acting compound Demecarium bromide 0.125–0.25% Ecothiophate iodide 0.03% Diisopropyl fluorophosphates 0.025–0.1%		15–25%	Same as direct-acting drugs

Local/systemic side effects
    Similar but more pronounced than with direct-acting compounds

Table 7. Hypertonic or osmotic agents

Compound	Mode of action	IOP reduction	Contraindications

Oral compound
  Glycerol
  Isosorbide
  Alcohol
	Dehydration and reduction in vitreous volume
	Posterior movement of the iris-lens plane with deepening of the anterior chamber
		15–20%	Cardiac or renal failure

Intravenous compound
  Mannitol
  Urea
		15–30%	

Side effects
    Nausea, vomiting, dehydration (special caution in diabetic patients)
    Increased diuresis, hyponatremia (if severe) may lead to lethargy, obtundation, seizure, coma
    Possible increase in blood glucose, acute oliguric renal failure, hypersensitivity reactions

caution in patients with slow or irregular heartbeat or congestive heart failure. Finally, adverse effects from the use of β-blockers include depression, impotence, and drowsiness. Two drops of 0.5% timolol equates to a 10-mg oral dose. This is not enough to cause symptoms in many patients, but unfortunately glaucoma and airway disease frequently coexist. For many years, β-blockers have been the most frequently used first-line and first-choice antiglaucoma medication, but they are replaced by prostaglandins in many countries now.

Carbonic Anhydrase Inhibitors

CAIs reduce IOP by inhibiting the ciliary epithelium and controlling aqueous formation. Acetazolamide and methazolamide are able to reduce IOP when taken orally. An IOP reduction of 30–40% can be expected. Systemic CAIs have been used since 1956. Methazolamide is given two times daily and acetazolamide four times daily. Acetazolamide is available as a slow-release formulation, which can be dosed twice a day.

Systemic CAIs can cause several side effects, including paresthesia of the lips, fingertips, and toes, fatigue, depression, kidney stones, anorexia, weight reduction, nausea, diarrhea, metabolic acidosis, agranulocytosis, aplastic anemia, and the Stevens-Johnsons syndrome.

Since 1994, a topical CAI has been available (fig. 7). An IOP reduction of 20% can be expected (fig. 6). Even though the adverse effects are much less compared to systemically administered CAIs, topical CAIs have some ocular adverse reactions, such as conjunctival allergy and hyperemia. Carbon anhydrase naturally exists in endothelial cells, and CAIs should be used with caution in patients with corneal endothelial disorders.

Sympathomimetic Drugs

α$_2$-Selective Adrenergic Receptor Agonists. α-Adrenergic agonists, more specifically the autoreceptors of α$_2$-neurons, are used in the treatment of glaucoma by decreasing the production of aqueous fluid by the ciliary bodies of the eye and also by increasing uveoscleral outflow. Sympathomimetic drugs like brimonidine and apraclonidine act on α$_2$-receptors and activate G-protein-coupled receptors, thereby reducing cAMP. In this way, the production of aqueous humor is reduced and uveoscleral outflow is increased. Brimonidine is able to reduce IOP by approximately 18–25% (fig. 6) and apraclonidine by 25–35% [13]. Approximately 45% of patients treated with apraclonidine show tachyphylaxis at the end of 6 months [4]. The recommended dosing frequency is three times per day.

It is contraindicated in infants, in whom it can cause serious systemic side effects. Allergic reactions frequently occur with this class of medication, especially with apraclonidine. Unfortunately, an allergy rate of 15–30% has been observed. Side effects may further include irregular heart rate, elevated blood pressure, headaches, blurred vision, fatigue, dry mouth, and redness in or around the eye. A randomized trial of the α$_2$-receptor agonist brimonidine versus the β-blocker timolol found a less likely visual field progression in patients treated with brimonidine compared to timolol, but a potential neuroprotective role of α$_2$-agonists in humans is still under debate.

Nonselective Adrenergic Agonists. Nonselective adrenergic agonists such as epinephrine and dipivefrin decrease aqueous humor production and may increase uveoscleral outflow. These drugs lower IOP by 15–20% on average (fig. 6). Nonselective adrenergic agonists are infrequently used today for the treatment of glaucoma or ocular hypertension; they have been replaced by the α$_2$-selective agonists mentioned above.

Parasympathomimetics or Cholinergic Agonists (Miotics)

Parasympathomimetic drugs are cholinergic agents that cause pupil constriction thereby increasing the rate of fluid drainage from the eye through the TM. Pilocarpine is the most commonly used cholinergic agonist. It is able to increase the outflow facility through conventional outflow pathways and lower IOP by 20–25% on average. It is less effective in eyes with dark irides. Pilocarpine gel is applied once a day and pilocarpine drops have to be given four times a day.

Adverse effects include miosis, induced accommodation, brow ache, myopic shift, further decrease in vision in patients with cataracts, visual field constriction due to the pupillary constriction, and reduced vision in darkness. An increased risk of retinal detachment (especially in patients with high myopia) and iritis has been noted. Overdosing miotics may cause excessive salivation and tearing, sweating, diarrhea, vomiting, and slowed heart rate.

Hypertonic or Osmotic Agents

Osmotic agents are an additional class of medications used to treat sudden (acute) forms of glaucoma where the eye pressure remains extremely high despite other treatments. These medications include isosorbide (Ismotic, p.o.) and mannitol (Osmitrol, i.v.). These medications must be used cautiously as they have significant side effects, including nausea, fluid accumulation in the heart and/or lungs (congestive heart failure and/or pulmonary edema), bleeding in the brain, and kidney problems. Their use is prohibited in patients with uncontrolled diabetes, and heart, kidney, or liver problems.

Role of Preservatives

Long-term topical glaucoma medications may cause and/or exacerbate preexisting ocular surface disease (OSD), such as dry eye, Meibomian gland dysfunction, and chronic allergy, which has a much higher prevalence in glaucoma patients than in the general population. OSD may follow chronic use of antiglaucoma medication and/or the preservative BAK. BAK, a quaternary ammonium compound, is the most frequently used preservative agent in eye drops, and its usage correlates well with the signs and symptoms of OSD. Such signs and symptoms can diminish if BAK-preserved drops are substituted with nonpreserved drops. An unwanted effect of BAK is a reduction in the success rate of filtering surgery [19–21].

In vitro studies suggest that alternative preservatives like Polyquad are significantly less toxic than BAK [22–26].

Other therapeutic possibilities are the use of preservative- or BAK-free medication; decreasing the number of preserved eye drops, i.e. by using fixed combinations; treating the ocular surface with unpreserved tear substitutes, and perform-

ing earlier laser treatment or surgery. Regarding OSD, four factors have to be considered: the active compound, the specific preservative, the ability of the patient to use single-dose preparations, and the patient's ocular surface.

The European Medicines Agency (EMEA) has suggested that the use of preservatives should be avoided in 'patients who do not tolerate eye drops with preservatives' and in those on long-term treatment, or to use a 'concentration at the minimum level consistent with satisfactory antimicrobial function in each individual preparation', with a specific indication to avoid mercury-containing preparations.

Not all patients are sensitive to preservatives and not all the local side effects observed with topical antiglaucoma medications are induced by preservatives.

Particular attention should be paid to glaucoma patients with preexisting OSD or those developing dry eye or ocular irritation over time. This can be done by careful assessment of redness of the eyelid margin, positive corneal and conjunctival fluorescein staining, or reduced tear break-up time.

Generic Intraocular Pressure-Lowering Topical Medications

By definition, a generic drug is identical to a brand name drug in dosage, strength, route of administration, performance characteristics, and intended use. For the purposes of drug approval, the interchangeability of a generic drug and the corresponding brand name drug is based on the criterion of 'essential similarity'. In ophthalmology, this concept is problematic, because it is difficult to prove 'essential similarity' in clinical studies. With systemic drugs, bioequivalence studies are performed using blood samples to determine whether the plasma concentration within certain limits equals the branded drug. With topical eye drops, such studies obviously cannot be performed.

Clinical studies are usually not required for generic approval in ophthalmology, and a 10% difference in the concentration of the active principle between the generic and the branded product is considered acceptable. Whereas the active principle is assumed to be equal, the adjuvants can vary considerably. This is a critical issue because different adjuvants may alter the viscosity, osmolarity, and pH of the eye drops, and, therefore, have an impact on both tolerability and corneal penetration.

Nevertheless, antiglaucoma generic drugs are currently prescribed at a large scale, as many drugs are becoming off patent. For latanoprost, the generic share is more than 65% in most European countries in 2014. To which degree these generics are similar in efficacy and tolerability is not well studied. Only few clinical studies have compared the effect of generic and brand IOP-lowering medications in glaucoma, with variable results depending on the type of generic drug [27, 28]. Other studies have shown a difference between the branded and the generic preparations concerning the size and amount of drops in the bottle, the structure of the bottle, and the bottle tips [29–31]. Safety issues with corneal epithelial disorders have also been described with generics due to an additional stabilizer compound [32]. When switching patients from branded to generic drugs, the IOP should be closely monitored.

How to Treat Glaucoma with Intraocular Pressure-Lowering Drugs
Start with Monotherapy
It is recommended to initiate the treatment with monotherapy (fig. 6, 9). Treatment is considered 'effective' when the achieved IOP reduction on treatment is comparable to the published average range for that drug in a similar population. According to a meta-analysis of randomized controlled trials, the highest reduction in IOP is obtained with prostaglandins, followed by nonselective β-blockers, α-adrenergic agonists, selective β-blockers, and, at last, topical CAIs [33].

It should be noted, however, that treatment effects depend on baseline IOP, with larger reductions in patients with higher pretreatment pressure levels. At low IOP values, medical and/or laser therapy have a smaller effect on IOP. Therefore, when evaluating the efficacy of a therapy or a drug it is important to consider the pretreatment baseline IOP [18].

If this initial therapy reduces IOP to the target and is well tolerated, therapy can be left unchanged, but the patient needs to be monitored with regular checking of endpoints.

Switching Monotherapy
If the target IOP has not been reached with monotherapy, then EGS recommends switching to another monotherapy before adding or combining.

Combination Therapy
If the target IOP has not been reached with monotherapy even after switching, then EGS recommends to add a new IOP-lowering drug, preferable as a fixed-combination eye drop. The options available today include prostaglandin analogs/β-blockers (prostaglandin and timolol), CAIs/β-blockers (dorzolamide or brinzolamide and timolol), and α_2-adrenergic agonists/β-blockers (brimonidine and timolol), and finally a combination of CAIs/α_2-adrenergic agonists (brinzolamide and brimonidine).

The benefit of fixed-combination eye drops is less exposure to preservatives and in many cases improved compliance.

Target Intraocular Pressure
Therapy in glaucoma management aims to lower IOP to slow the rate of visual field deterioration.

Target IOP is the upper limit of the IOP estimated to be compatible with a rate of progression sufficiently slow to maintain vision-related quality of life in the expected lifetime of the patient. It should be reevaluated regularly and, additionally, when progression of disease is identified, or when ocular or systemic comorbidities develop.

There is no single target IOP level that is appropriate for every patient, so the target IOP

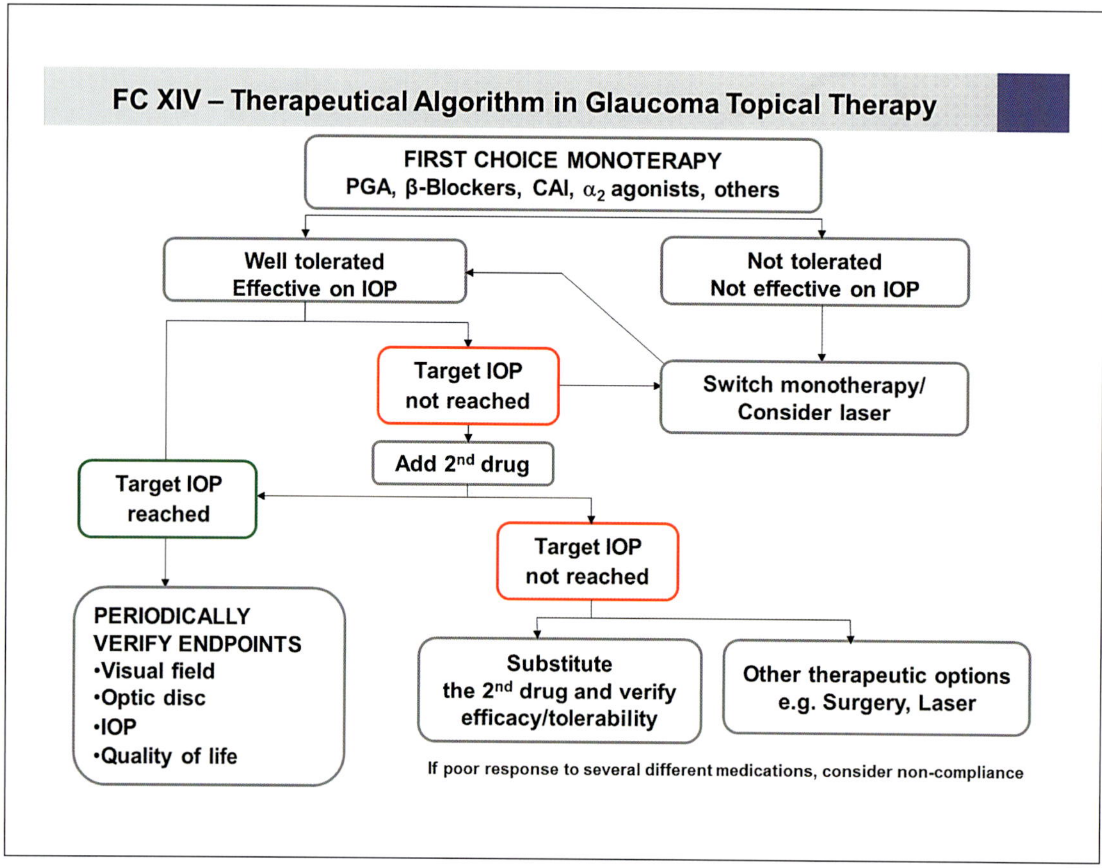

Fig. 9. Therapeutic algorithm in glaucoma topical therapy. PGA = Prostaglandin analog. Reprinted with permission from the European Glaucoma Society (EGS Guidelines 2014).

needs to be estimated separately for each eye in every patient (fig. 7–9).

General Recommendations in Medical Glaucoma Therapy

- Monotherapy is the first choice when initiating therapy.
- Baseline IOP should be considered when evaluating the efficacy of a therapy.
- Fixed-combination therapy should be considered when patients fail to achieve their individualized IOP targets with monotherapy.
- The prescription of more than two bottles of IOP-lowering eye drops for simultaneous use should be avoided as it can lead to noncompliance.
- Fixed-combination preparations may be preferable to the use of separate instillation of two agents.
- However, fixed-combination therapies are not first-line medications and they are only indicated in patients who need adjunctive therapy, when IOP is not sufficiently controlled by monotherapy.
- Ocular surface should be evaluated and considered in the clinical management of glaucoma patients. In case of OSD, preservative-free formulations should be considered.

Table 8. Targets for new treatment strategies in the management of glaucoma (reprinted with permission from Kolko [34])

IOP-lowering strategies	Neuroprotective strategies	Neuroregenerative strategies
Increasing TM outflow	*Excitotoxicity*	*Cell repair*
ROCK	NMDA antagonists (memantine)	Inflammatory stimulation (CNTF)
Endothelin-1	Modulation of Müller cells	Gene therapy (Nogo receptor interference)
Nitric oxide	*Oxidative stress*	*Surgical approaches*
TGF-β	Antioxidants (α-tocopherol)	Lens injury
CTGF	Ginkgo biloba	*Stem cell therapy*
Adenosine	*Mitochondrial dysfunction*	CNTF-secreting retinal pigment epithelial cells
Angiopoietin-like-7 molecules	Mitochondrial-targeted antioxidants (Q10)	
Cannabinoids	*Inflammation/abnormal immune responses*	
Cochlin	TNF-α	
Latrunculins	Biological response modifiers (etanercept)	
Melatonin	Agmatine	
Ghrelin	Modulation of T-cell reaction (Cop-1)	
Increasing uveoscleral outflow	Modulation of PLA$_2$-induced inflammation	
Angiotensin II	*Protein misfolding*	
Serotonin	Agents targeting amyloid β	
Ghrelin	Heat shock proteins	
Cannabinoids	*Glial cell modulation*	
Decreasing aqueous humor production	TGF-β, CNTF, PDGF	
Forskolin	*Other pathways*	
Serotonin	Estradiol	
Cannabinoids	Statins	
Angiotensin II	Erythropoietin	

CTGF = Connective tissue growth factor; PDGF = platelet-derived growth factor; PLA$_2$ = phospholipase A$_2$; TGF = transforming growth factor.

- Generic drops can differ from brand drops, and it may be necessary to monitor patients more closely after switching.
- During pregnancy, the potential risks of continuing antiglaucoma medications to the fetus (and neonate) must be balanced against the risk of vision loss in the mother.

Mechanisms of Glaucoma Medications: Future Treatment

This part is based upon open source reviews by Rocha-Sousa et al. [6] and Kolko [34].

New drugs are now entering the clinic, along with new ways to deliver them. There is growing consensus that the future of glaucoma management will be based more on the optic nerve pathway from the retina to the visual cortex and not strictly limited to improving outflow or reducing inflow. But still, many future IOP-lowering options will be developed (tables 8, 9).

Lowering Intraocular Pressure (Future Options)
Increasing Trabecular Meshwork Outflow

IOP can be lowered by ρ-associated kinase (ROCK) inhibitors, endothelin-1, and nitric oxide, for example.

ρ-Associated Kinase Inhibitors. ROCK inhibitors are thought to enhance aqueous drainage by acting on the actin cytoskeleton and cellular motility in the TM, Schlemm's canal, and in the cili-

Table 9. New therapeutic targets for IOP lowering and possible mechanisms of action (reprinted from Rocha-Sousa et al. [6])

Pathways	Mechanisms of action
ρ-Kinase	Modulation may increase TM outflow by modulation of contractility/TM cytoskeleton disruption
Endothelin-1	Modulation may increase TM outflow by modulation of contractility/TM cytoskeleton disruption
Transforming growth factor-β	Modulation may increase TM outflow by remodeling extracellular matrix and/or by modulation of contractility/TM cytoskeleton disruption
Connective tissue growth factor	Modulation may increase TM outflow by remodeling extracellular matrix
Nitric oxide	Modulation may increase TM outflow by modulation of TM cell contractility
Angiopoietin-like molecules	Modulation may increase TM outflow by remodeling extracellular matrix
Adenosine	Modulation may increase TM outflow by remodeling extracellular matrix
Latrunculins	Modulation may increase TM outflow by modulation of contractility/TM cytoskeleton disruption
Cochlin	Modulation may increase TM outflow by potential mechanosensing mechanisms
Cannabinoids	Modulation may decrease AH production, and/or may increase TM outflow (by increasing the dimensions of Schlemm's canal and/or by remodeling extracellular matrix) and/or may increase uveoscleral outflow
Melatonin	Modulation may increase TM outflow trough cholinergic and noradrenergic systems
Ghrelin	Modulation may increase TM outflow and/or uveoscleral outflow
Angiotensin II	Modulation may increase uveoscleral outflow and/or decrease AH production
Serotonin	Modulation may increase uveoscleral outflow and decrease AH production
Forskolin	Modulation may decrease AH production

AH = Aqueous humor.

ary muscle. These drugs appear to lower IOP by decreasing resistance to aqueous outflow by cellular relaxation in the TM.

Endothelin-1. Endothelin-1 is another TM modulator, and a significant correlation has been found between IOP and endothelin-1.

Nitric Oxide. Nitric oxide has been implicated in more mechanisms related to glaucoma such as autoregulation of RGC survival and death, and low-grade inflammation [35]. Nitric oxide agonists also induce relaxation of TM cells and thereby increase outflow [36, 37].

Increasing Uveoscleral Outflow
Uveoscleral outflow can be increased by angiotensin II for example.

Angiotensin II. Compounds that increase angiotensin-converting enzyme 2 (ACE2) activity and further the formation of angiotensin (1–7) are new options as anti-glaucomatous drugs in addition to classical ACE inhibitors and angiotensin I receptor blockers.

Other New Targets to Increase Uveoscleral Outflow. In addition to angiotensin II treatment, targets such as serotonin, ghrelin, and cannabinoids [38] have also been suggested as potential drugs to increase uveoscleral outflow (fig. 10). A major problem with *marijuana* for glaucoma is that the half-life of the drug itself is very short, usually 3–4 h. Most current drugs that are used for glaucoma are taken one or two times per day; a drug needing to be taken 6–8 times a day is not patient friendly and would likely lead to decreased adherence. Unsurprisingly, the American Glaucoma Society declared that marijuana is not recommended for the treatment of glaucoma.

Decreasing Aqueous Humor Production
Examples are forskolin, serotonin, cannabinoids, and angiotensin II.

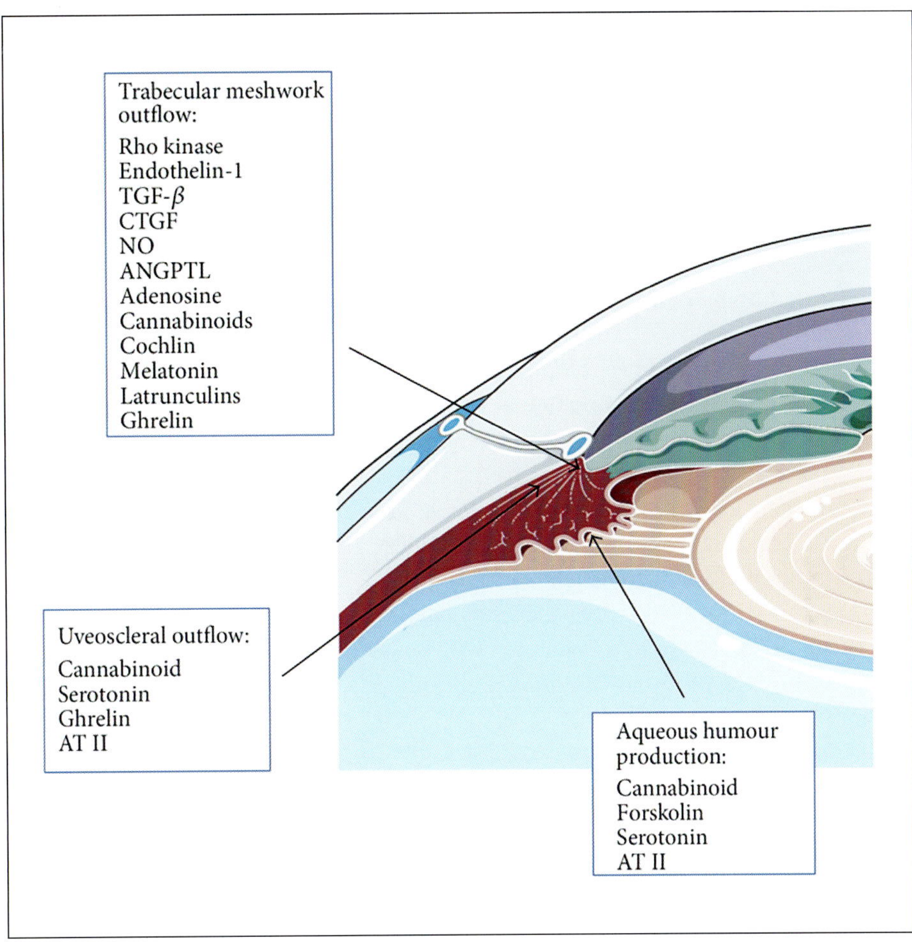

Fig. 10. New therapeutic targets that lower IOP. Mechanisms of action are indicated (Rocha-Sousa et al. [6]). ANGPTL = Angiopoietin-like molecules; AT II = angiotensin II; CTGF = connective tissue growth factor; NO = nitric oxide. Reprinted from Rocha-Sousa et al. [6].

Non-Intraocular Pressure-Lowering Strategies
Lowering IOP remains the only proven method to prevent the development or to slow the progression of glaucomatous optic neuropathy. Interestingly, a significant proportion of the treatment groups in the Early Manifest Glaucoma Trial [3], the Collaborative Initial Glaucoma Treatment Study [4], and the Collaborative Normal-Tension Glaucoma Study [39] experienced glaucomatous progression despite achieving the targeted decrease in IOP.

Although the cause of disease progression despite seemingly adequate IOP lowering is likely multifactorial, non-IOP-lowering strategies need to come into consideration.

Neuroprotective Strategies
Neuroprotection can be defined as a 'therapeutic approach' aiming to directly prevent or significantly hinder neuronal cell damage. Since glaucoma patients can continue deteriorating in spite of an apparently well-controlled IOP, the need for

effective non-IOP-related treatments is widely acknowledged. Several compounds have been neuroprotectant in preclinical studies. Only two have reached large-scale clinical trials: a large long-term randomized controlled trial using an NMDA antagonist, *memantine*, was analyzed in 2008 with negative results. More recently, the results from a multicenter randomized controlled trial of 178 adults with low-pressure glaucoma (Low-Pressure Glaucoma Treatment Study) tested whether the α₂-adrenergic agonist *brimonidine* had neuroprotective properties by slowing the rate of visual field deterioration in subjects with normal-pressure glaucoma. Fewer patients on brimonidine worsened over time compared with those receiving timolol [11]. This occurred despite similar decreases in IOP with the two drugs. However, the results of this study need to be confirmed before they can be accepted as hard evidence [12, 40, 41]. No direct comparison has been done with other substances such as prostaglandins.

In order to simplify the complexity of the proposed new neuroprotective treatment strategies, these can be grouped into targets that interfere with excitotoxicity, oxidative stress, mitochondrial dysfunction, inflammation/abnormal immune responses, protein misfolding, and glial cell modulation. Most targets will interfere with more pathways.

Excitotoxicity. Excitotoxicity refers to the pathological process by which neurons are damaged by the overactivation of glutamate receptors. In glaucoma, the initial insult to RGCs has been suggested to lead to elevated levels of extracellular glutamate resulting in a massive influx of calcium into the neurons, thereby causing glutamate-mediated RGC death. Strategies to modify glutamate-induced neurotoxicity have been widely explored, and, in particular, the NMDA antagonist memantine has been shown to be a highly effective neuroprotective agent in both acute and chronic animal models of RGC death [42, 43]. In a well-known *memantine* clinical trial, no significant benefit was found in the memantine-treated group compared to the patients receiving placebo

[44]. The largest study examined the ability of *memantine* to decrease the progression of glaucoma in two parallel trials of more than 2,000 patients. The results of the study have not been published, but press releases from Allergan, the pharmaceutical company that funded the study, indicated that the primary outcome measure in each of the trials was not met. There are no published data on specific results from this study, including other outcome measures and subgroup analyses.

Oxidative Stress. Oxidative stress reflects an imbalance between the production of reactive oxygen species and the ability of cells to readily detoxify the reactive intermediates or to repair the resulting damage. Significant evidence has shown that oxidative stress plays a role in RGC death in glaucoma, and the concept of antioxidants as a neuroprotective treatment strategy is widely accepted [45–49]. Among the most studied antioxidants, vitamin E (α-tocopherol) and gingko biloba have been shown to ameliorate NMDA-induced RGC death. Vitamin E acts as a scavenger of peroxyl radicals. Although some studies have suggested a decreased rate of glaucomatous progression in patients receiving vitamin E, the long-term results are still lacking.

Gingko biloba is an extract from *Ginkgo biloba* leaves. It increases blood flow and has been shown to have a free radical scavenger property. In addition, gingko biloba has been shown to interfere with glutamate signaling and to preserve mitochondrial metabolism. The precise mechanism by which gingko biloba interferes with RGC homeostasis is still not fully understood, but the studied literature on gingko biloba is in favor of a possible beneficial effect on RGC survival [50, 51].

Mitochondrial Dysfunction. In line with the role of oxidative stress in the pathogenesis of glaucoma, increasing evidence points to a mitochondrial dysfunction in glaucoma. Among mitochondrial-targeted antioxidants, *coenzyme Q10* is one of the most studied targets, and, in animal models, Q10 protects RGCs after ischemia [52, 53] and oxidative stress [33]. To date, no human clinical trials have been published on the use of Q10 in glaucoma.

Inflammation/Abnormal Immune Responses. It is widely accepted that glaucomatous neurodegeneration comes with an activation of glial cells and accompanying production of proinflammatory cytokines, such as tumor necrosis factor (TNF)-α. The inflammatory process in glaucoma has been found to be associated with proinflammatory activities mediated in part by T-cell activity. It has been shown experimentally that glutamate injections into the eye result in T-cell reactions, and, in this aspect, Cop-1 immunization has shown some protection against RGC death.

Glial Cell Modulation. Much attention has been given to RGC maintenance in the search for new treatment targets in glaucoma. However, it is clear that the surrounding cells tightly regulate RGC homeostasis. Hence, in the nonmyelinated region of RGCs, Müller cells and astrocytes (macroglial cells) are the major glial cells to provide support, as well as to create the interface between RGCs and blood vessels. They remove excess glutamate from the synapse thereby preventing excitotoxicity, and help to maintain ion homeostasis and extracellular pH.

Other Pathways. Considerable evidence exists on estrogen as a neuroprotective drug, and a recent study has provided strong evidence that topical estrogen drops are neuroprotective in a rodent model of glaucoma. Other suggested drugs to prevent glaucomatous damage are statins. Hence, long-term use of statins has been shown to be associated with a reduced risk of glaucoma. Finally, the glycoprotein erythropoietin has been suggested to be a potential therapeutic neuroprotectant in glaucoma.

Neuroregenerative Strategies

Growing evidence suggests cell repair or cell replacement therapy as a new treatment approach. Within the potential group of cell repair treatment strategies, axonal growth has become a target for investigation. Furthermore, gene therapy and surgical approaches to enhance regenerative capacity of RGCs have been suggested. Finally, stem cells hold great promise for neurodegenerative disorders such as glaucoma.

Cell Repair or Gene Therapy. Although the critical first step in the treatment of glaucoma is enhancing RGC survival, a significant number of patients will be diagnosed at a later stage at which their axons have already been injured. In these cases, preventing apoptosis will not be sufficient, and the ideal therapies should encourage axon regeneration to rebuild connections from the RGCs to the brain. In this aspect, more molecules have been shown to possess regenerative properties due to their inflammatory stimulation. Among these, ciliary neurotrophic factor (CNTF) has been shown to induce axonal growth and thereby suggested to provide a new neuroregenerative approach [54, 55].

Surgical Approaches for Neuroregeneration. Penetrating injury as well as lens injury has been suggested to result in the release of low-grade inflammatory molecules, which secondarily leads to axonal regeneration. In order to consider this strategy in humans, a number of issues would have to be considered, including rapid formation of cataract and infection, for example. Hence, pursuing the molecular basis of the effect may prove more realistic for translation to human glaucoma treatment.

Stem Cell Therapy. Stem cell therapy holds great promise for neurodegenerative diseases, and emerging studies try to identify the use of stem cells in experimental glaucoma. Substantial evidence has correlated neurotrophic factor deprivation with RGC death and new therapies aim to supplement these. To avoid repeated injections of growth factors, cell-based delivery of neurotrophic factors has been proposed. In this matter, an ongoing phase-I clinical trial for glaucoma is using genetically modified CNTF-secreting retinal pigment epithelial cells.

Stem Cell Transplantation. In addition, transplantation of mesenchymal stem cells (MSC) has been suggested, since these produce neurotrophic factors [56]. Furthermore, intracranial human umbilical cord blood MSC transplantation has been shown to protect RGC and to induce axonal regeneration [57]. Overall, the neuroprotective and neuroregenerative effect of MSCs on RGC survival is evident, and, currently, a clinical trial using bone marrow-derived MSCs on glaucoma is in process. The outcome of this study is expected in 2017.

Improved Optic Nerve Perfusion

Although the cause of disease progression despite seemingly adequate IOP lowering is likely multifactorial, abnormalities in ocular perfusion have become a prime consideration. Vascular risk factors for glaucomatous progression implicate abnormal or insufficient blood flow to the optic nerve as a likely contributor to the disease process [58, 59].

Decreased blood flow parameters in the retrobulbar, retinal, ONH, and choroidal circulations have all been shown to correlate with visual field defects. In addition, morphologic changes in the retina, ONH, and choroid are associated with altered blood flow. These findings, along with concepts such as fluctuations in perfusion, promote the possibility of ischemic injury in open-angle glaucoma.

Low ocular perfusion pressure (OPP) may be used to determine whether abnormal microvascular flow is likely to occur at the level of the optic nerve. OPP is defined as the mean arterial pressure minus the IOP. Epidemiologic studies have identified low OPP as an independent risk factor for the development and progression of glaucoma [60, 61].

In preliminary animal studies, ρ-kinase inhibitors have been shown to improve optic nerve blood flow, presumably via relaxation of the vascular endothelial smooth muscle. These agents are not yet commercially available but are in clinical trials for approval by the FDA.

Topical ρ-kinase inhibitors may also prove to be a therapeutic option. Clinicians' ability to diagnose and treat blood flow abnormalities in the ONH may allow them to decrease the risk of glaucomatous progression in individuals with an IOP-independent component to their disease process.

So far, we have no evidence of potential therapies related to ocular blood flow and glaucoma care.

Key Issues in Improved Optic Nerve Perfusion [62]

- IOP is the only known treatable risk factor to decrease progression of open-angle glaucoma.
- Sufficient evidence exists from clinical trials to conclude that ocular blood flow deficits are associated with glaucoma.
- Recent evidence has shown that blood flow deficits lead to structural and functional damage.
- In large population trials, decreased OPP has been associated with the prevalence and progression of glaucoma.
- Greater fluctuations in ocular blood flow and OPP have been shown to be associated with the development of glaucoma and progression of visual field loss.
- Currently, there is insufficient evidence to conclude that insufficient blood flow directly causes glaucoma progression.
- Future studies will look at glaucoma progression as it relates to ocular blood flow parameters in longitudinal studies involving an increased number of patients and more standardized methods.
- Assessment of blood flow will need to move away from surrogate measures of blood flow and more towards measurement of oxygenation and metabolism of ocular tissues.

General Health Issues in Glaucoma

Glaucoma is still a leading cause of blindness in Europe. A considerable percentage of glaucoma patients become blind in both eyes or encounter serious field loss in both eyes [1, 63, 64]. Major risk factors for glaucoma blindness are the severity of the disease at presentation and life expectancy [1, 2]. A 60-year-old patient with bilateral moderate visual function damage at diagnosis has a greater risk of blindness than an 85-year-old patient with a similar amount of damage. Similarly, a young patient with mild bilateral damage is at much larger risk of disability in his lifetime than an 80-year-old patient with moderate unilateral disease Thus, treatment must be individualized to the needs and rate of progression of each patient. The risk of ever encountering loss of quality of life from glaucoma should determine target pressure, intensity of treatment, and frequency of follow-up.

Thus, patients with severe functional loss or younger patients with manifest disease should have more aggressive treatment and closer follow-up than patients with little or no risk, e.g. very old patients with early visual field loss or unilateral disease. Glaucoma suspects, e.g. patients with elevated IOP and otherwise normal findings, have even smaller risks.

In most patients with advanced glaucoma and reasonable life expectancy, aggressive IOP-lowering treatment might be recommended [65, 66]. Very old patients with mild function loss, relatively low IOP levels, and significant health problems might prefer being followed without treatment. When treatment options are discussed with a patient, his general health status and personal preferences must be considered and respected. It is also important to ensure that patients are able to comply and persist with therapy.

The goal of glaucoma treatment is to maintain the patient's visual function and related quality of life at a sustainable cost. The cost of treatment in terms of inconvenience and side effects as well as financial implications for the individual and society requires careful evaluation. Quality of life is closely linked with visual function and, overall, patients with early to moderate glaucoma damage have good visual function and modest reduction in quality of life, while quality of life is considerably reduced if *both* eyes have advanced visual function loss.

Individualized glaucoma treatment aims at providing glaucoma management tailored to the individual needs of the patient; patients with severe functional loss or younger patients with manifest disease should have more aggressive treatment and closer follow-up than patients with little or no risk, e.g. patients with ocular hypertension or elderly patients with mild field loss and low IOP levels [61, 67–70].

Conclusion

- IOP lowering is the only proven therapy for glaucoma at present.
- Neuroprotection may be clinically useful (based on one trial), but this needs to be confirmed.
- So far, we have no evidence of potential therapies related to ocular blood flow and glaucoma care.
- There is insufficient evidence to support the use of acupuncture, vitamins, minerals, or herbal medicines like marijuana for treating glaucoma.

References

1 Peters D, Bengtsson B, Heijl A: Factors associated with lifetime risk of open-angle glaucoma blindness. Acta Ophthalmol 2014;92:421–425

2 Martus P, Stroux A, Budde WM, et al: Predictive factors for progressive optic nerve damage in various types of chronic open-angle glaucoma. Am J Ophthalmol 2005;139:999–1009.

3 Heijl A, Leske MC, Bengtsson B, et al: Reduction of intraocular pressure and glaucoma progression: results from the Early Manifest Glaucoma Trial. Arch Ophthalmol 2002;120:1268–1279.

4 Lichter PR, Musch DC, Gillespie BW, et al: Interim clinical outcomes in the Collaborative Initial Glaucoma Treatment Study comparing initial treatment randomized to medications or surgery. Ophthalmology 2001;108:1943–1953.

5   The Glaucoma Laser Trial (GLT): 6. Treatment group differences in visual field changes. Glaucoma Laser Trial Research Group. Am J Ophthalmol 1995; 120:10–22.

6   Rocha-Sousa A, Rodrigues-Araújo J, Gouveia P, et al: New therapeutic targets for intraocular pressure lowering. ISRN Ophthalmol 2013;2013:261386.

7   Gherghel D, Orgul S, Gugleta K, et al: Relationship between ocular perfusion pressure and retrobulbar blood flow in patients with glaucoma with progressive damage. Am J Ophthalmol 2000;130: 597–605.

8   Flammer J, Orgul S, Costa VP, et al: The impact of ocular blood flow in glaucoma. Prog Retin Eye Res 2002;21:359–393.

9   Grieshaber MC, Mozaffarieh M, Flammer J: What is the link between vascular dysregulation and glaucoma? Surv Ophthalmol 2007;52(suppl 2):S144–S154.

10 Tielsch JM, Katz J, Sommer A, et al: Hypertension, perfusion pressure, and primary open-angle glaucoma. A population-based assessment. Arch Ophthalmol 1995;113:216–221.

11 Krupin T, Liebmann JM, Greenfield DS, et al: A randomized trial of brimonidine versus timolol in preserving visual function: results from the Low-Pressure Glaucoma Treatment Study. Am J Ophthalmol 2011;151:671–681.

12 Sena DF, Lindsley K: Neuroprotection for treatment of glaucoma in adults. The Cochrane Database Syst Rev 2013; 2:CD006539.

13 Kass MA, Heuer DK, Higginbotham EJ, et al: The Ocular Hypertension Treatment Study: a randomized trial determines that topical ocular hypotensive medication delays or prevents the onset of primary open-angle glaucoma. Arch Ophthalmol 2002;120:701–713; discussion 829–830.

14 Miglior S, Zeyen T, Pfeiffer N, et al: Results of the European Glaucoma Prevention Study. Ophthalmology 2005;112: 366–375.

15 Boland MV, Ervin AM, Friedman DS, et al: Comparative effectiveness of treatments for open-angle glaucoma: a systematic review for the U.S. Preventive Services Task Force. Ann Intern Med 2013;158:271–279.

16 Leske MC, Heijl A, Hussein M, et al: Factors for glaucoma progression and the effect of treatment: the early manifest glaucoma trial. Arch Ophthalmol 2003;121:48–56.

17 Chauhan BC, Mikelberg FS, Balaszi AG, et al: Canadian Glaucoma Study. 2. Risk factors for the progression of open-angle glaucoma. Arch Ophthalmol 2008;126: 1030–1036.

18 van der Valk R, Webers CA, Schouten JS, et al: Intraocular pressure-lowering effects of all commonly used glaucoma drugs: a meta-analysis of randomized clinical trials. Ophthalmology 2005;112: 1177–1185.

19 Thieme H, van der Velden KK: Preservatives from the perspective of glaucoma surgery (in German). Ophthalmologe 2012;109:1073–1076.

20 Boimer C, Birt CM: Preservative exposure and surgical outcomes in glaucoma patients: the PESO Study. J Glaucoma 2013;22:730–735.

21 Batra R, Tailor R, Mohamed S: Ocular surface disease exacerbated glaucoma: optimizing the ocular surface improves intraocular pressure control. J Glaucoma 2014;23:56–60.

22 Ammar DA, Noecker RJ, Kahook MY: Effects of benzalkonium chloride-preserved, polyquad-preserved, and sofZia-preserved topical glaucoma medications on human ocular epithelial cells. Adv Ther 2010;27:837–845.

23 Ammar DA, Noecker RJ, Kahook MY: Effects of benzalkonium chloride- and polyquad-preserved combination glaucoma medications on cultured human ocular surface cells. Adv Ther 2011;28: 501–510.

24 Brignole-Baudouin F, Riancho L, Liang H, et al: In vitro comparative toxicology of Polyquad-preserved and benzalkonium chloride-preserved travoprost/timolol fixed combination and latanoprost/timolol fixed combination. J Ocul Pharmacol Ther 2011;27:273–280.

25 Xu M, Sivak JG, McCanna DJ: Comparison of the effects of ophthalmic solutions on human corneal epithelial cells using fluorescent dyes. J Ocul Pharmacol Ther 2013;29:794–802.

26 Noecker R: Effects of common ophthalmic preservatives on ocular health. Adv Ther 2001;18:205–215.

27 Allaire C, Dietrich A, Allmeier H, et al: Latanoprost 0.005% test formulation is as effective as Xalatan® in patients with ocular hypertension and primary open-angle glaucoma. Eur J Ophthalmol 2012; 22:19–27.

28 Narayanaswamy A, Neog A, Baskaran M, et al: A randomized, crossover, open label pilot study to evaluate the efficacy and safety of Xalatan in comparison with generic latanoprost (Latoprost) in subjects with primary open angle glaucoma or ocular hypertension. Indian J Ophthalmol 2007;55:127–131.

29 Lu D, Hong L, Xu X, et al: Chemical analysis of branded latanoprost 0.005% compared with commercially available latanoprost formulations. ARVO Meeting Abstracts 2010;51:3162.

30 Brian S, Jayat C, Desmis A, Garrigue J-S: Pharmaceutical evaluation of the quality and delivered dose of US latanoprost generics. ARVO Meeting Abstracts 2012;53:5103.

31 Joag M, Thirumurthy V, Jha B, et al: Comparative evaluation of physical properties of 3 commercially available generic brands of latanoprost with Xalatan. ARVO Meeting Abstracts 2012;53:5096.

32 Mammo ZN, Flanagan JG, James DF, Trope GE: Generic versus brand-name North American topical glaucoma drops. Can J Ophthalmol 2012;47:55–61.

33 Nakajima Y, Inokuchi Y, Nishi M, Shimazawa M, Otsubo K, Hara H: Coenzyme Q10 protects retinal cells against oxidative stress in vitro and in vivo. Brain Res 2008;1226:226–233.

34 Kolko M: Present and new treatment strategies in the management of glaucoma. Open Ophthalmol J 2015;9:89–100.

35 Vohra R, Tsai JC, Kolko M: The role of inflammation in the pathogenesis of glaucoma. Surv Ophthalmol 2013;58: 311–320.

36 Nathanson JA, McKee M: Identification of an extensive system of nitric oxide-producing cells in the ciliary muscle and outflow pathway of the human eye. Invest Ophthalmol Vis Sci 1995;36:1765–1773.

37 Wiederholt M, Thieme H, Stumpff F: The regulation of trabecular meshwork and ciliary muscle contractility. Prog Retin Eye Res 2000;19:271–295.

38 Pinar-Sueiro S, Rodríguez-Puertas R, Vecino E: Cannabinoid applications in glaucoma (in Spanish). Arch Soc Esp Oftalmol 2011;86:16–23.

39 Collaborative Normal-Tension Glaucoma Study Group. Comparison of glaucomatous progression between untreated patients with normal-tension glaucoma and patients with therapeutically reduced intraocular pressures. Am J Ophthalmol 1998;126:487–497.

40 Baltmr A, Duggan J, Nizari S, et al: Neuroprotection in glaucoma – is there a future role? Exp Eye Res 2010;91:554–566.

41 Cordeiro MF, Levin LA: Clinical evidence for neuroprotection in glaucoma. Am J Ophthalmol 2011;152:715–716.

42 Hare WA, WoldeMussie E, Lai RK, Ton H, Ruiz G, Chun T, Wheeler L: Efficacy and safety of memantine treatment for reduction of changes associated with experimental glaucoma in monkey. I. Functional measures. Invest Ophthalmol Vis Sci 2004;45:2625–2639.

43 Miguel-Hidalgo JJ, Alvarez XA, Cacabelos R, Quack G: Neuroprotection by memantine against neurodegeneration induced by beta-amyloid (1–40). Brain Res 2002;958:210–221.

44 Osborne NN: Recent clinical findings with memantine should not mean that the idea of neuroprotection in glaucoma is abandoned. Acta Ophthalmol 2009; 87:450–454.

45 Feilchenfeld Z, Yücel YH, Gupta N: Oxidative injury to blood vessels and glia of the pre-laminar optic nerve head in human glaucoma. Exp Eye Res 2008;87: 409–414.

46 Javadiyan S, Burdon KP, Whiting MJ, Abhary S, Straga T, Hewitt AW, Mills RA, Craig JE: Elevation of serum asymmetrical and symmetrical dimethylarginine in patients with advanced glaucoma. Invest Ophthalmol Vis Sci 2012;53: 1923–1927.

47 Ko M-L, Peng P-H, Ma M-C, Ritch R, Chen C-F: Dynamic changes in reactive oxygen species and antioxidant levels in retinas in experimental glaucoma. Free Radic Biol Med 2005;39:365–373.

48 Moreno MC, Campanelli J, Sande P, Sánez DA, Keller Sarmiento MI, Rosenstein RE: Retinal oxidative stress induced by high intraocular pressure. Free Radic Biol Med 2004;37:803–812.

49 Tezel G, Yang X, Cai J: Proteomic identification of oxidatively modified retinal proteins in a chronic pressure-induced rat model of glaucoma. Invest Ophthalmol Vis Sci 2005;46:3177–3187.

50 Cybulska-Heinrich AK, Mozaffarieh M, Flammer J: Ginkgo biloba: an adjuvant therapy for progressive normal and high tension glaucoma. Mol Vis 2012;18: 390–402.

51 Lee J, Sohn SW, Kee C: Effect of ginkgo biloba extract on visual field progression in normal tension glaucoma. J Glaucoma 2013;22:780–784.

52 Nucci C, Tartaglione R, Cerulli A, Mancino R, Spanò A, Cavaliere F, Rombolà L, Bagetta G, Corasaniti MT, Morrone LA: Retinal damage caused by high intraocular pressure-induced transient ischemia is prevented by coenzyme Q10 in rat. Int Rev Neurobiol 2007;82:397–406.

53 Russo R, Cavaliere F, Rombolà L, Gliozzi M, Cerulli A, Nucci C, Fazzi E, Bagetta G, Corasaniti MT, Morrone LA: Rational basis for the development of coenzyme Q10 as a neurotherapeutic agent for retinal protection. Prog Brain Res 2008;173: 575–582.

54 Leibinger M, Andreadaki A, Fischer D: Role of mTOR in neuroprotection and axon regeneration after inflammatory stimulation. Neurobiol Dis 2012;46: 314–324.

55 Jo SA, Wang E, Benowitz LI: Ciliary neurotrophic factor is an axogenesis factor for retinal ganglion cells. Neuroscience 1999;89:579–591.

56 Johnson TV, Bull ND, Hunt DP, Marina N, Tomarev SI, Martin KR: Neuroprotective effects of intravitreal mesenchymal stem cell transplantation in experimental glaucoma. Invest Ophthalmol Vis Sci 2010;51:2051–2059.

57 Zwart I, Hill AJ, Al-Allaf F, Shah M, Girdlestone J, Sanusi AB, Mehmet H, Navarrete R, Navarrete C, Jen LS: Umbilical cord blood mesenchymal stromal cells are neuroprotective and promote regeneration in a rat optic tract model. Exp Neurol 2009;216:439–448.

58 Drance S, Anderson DR, Schulzer M: Collaborative Normal-Tension Glaucoma Study Group. Risk factors for progression of visual field abnormalities in normal-tension glaucoma. Am J Ophthalmol 2001;131:699–708.

59 Bonomi L, Marchini G, Marraffa M, et al: Vascular risk factors for primary open-angle glaucoma: the Egna-Neumarkt Study. Ophthalmology 2000;107: 1287–1293.

60 Leske MC, Wu SY, Hennis A, et al: Risk factors for incident open-angle glaucoma: the Barbados Eye Studies. Ophthalmology 2008;115:85–93.

61 Leske MC, Heijl A, Hyman L, et al: Predictors of long-term progression in the Early Manifest Glaucoma Trial. Ophthalmology 2007;114:1965–1972.

62 Siesky BA, Harris A, Amireskandari A, Marek B: Glaucoma and ocular blood flow: an anatomical perspective. Expert Rev Ophthalmol 2012;7:325–340.

63 Cedrone C, Nucci C, Scuderi G, et al: Prevalence of blindness and low vision in an Italian population: a comparison with other European studies. Eye (Lond) 2006;20:661–667.

64 Forsman E, Kivela T, Vesti E: Lifetime visual disability in open-angle glaucoma and ocular hypertension. J Glaucoma 2007;16:313–319.

65 The Advanced Glaucoma Intervention Study (AGIS): 7. The relationship between control of intraocular pressure and visual field deterioration. The AGIS Investigators. Am J Ophthalmol 2000; 130:429–440.

66 AGIS Investigators: The Advanced Glaucoma Intervention Study (AGIS): 12. Baseline risk factors for sustained loss of visual field and visual acuity in patients with advanced glaucoma. Am J Ophthalmol 2002;134:499–512.

67 Broman AT, Quigley HA, West SK, et al: Estimating the rate of progressive visual field damage in those with open-angle glaucoma, from cross-sectional data. Invest Ophthalmol Vis Sci 2008;49:66–76.

68 Chauhan BC, Garway-Heath DF, Goni FJ, et al: Practical recommendations for measuring rates of visual field change in glaucoma. Br J Ophthalmol 2008;92: 569–573.

69 Bengtsson B, Heijl A: A visual field index for calculation of glaucoma rate of progression. Am J Ophthalmol 2008; 145:343–353.

70 Heijl A, Bengtsson B, Chauhan BC, et al: A comparison of visual field progression criteria of 3 major glaucoma trials in early manifest glaucoma trial patients. Ophthalmology 2008;115:1557–1565.

Prof. Dr. John Thygesen
Department of Ophthalmology, Rigshospitalet
Copenhagen University Hospital, Nordre Ringvej 57
DK–2600 Glostrup (Denmark)
E-Mail john.thygesen@regionh.dk

Traverso CE, Stalmans I, Topouzis F, Bagnasco L (eds): Glaucoma.
ESASO Course Series. Basel, Karger, 2016, vol 8, pp 76–90 (DOI: 10.1159/000446138)

Laser Treatment in Glaucoma

Barbara Cvenkel

Department of Ophthalmology, University Medical Center Ljubljana, and Medical Faculty, University of
Ljubljana, Ljubljana, Slovenia

Abstract

In glaucoma patients, lasers are used to increase aqueous
humor outflow, treat internal block of aqueous flow, and
reduce aqueous humor production. The indications, techniques, and efficacy of various traditional glaucoma laser
procedures such as argon laser trabeculoplasty (ALT), iridoplasty, laser peripheral iridotomy, and cyclophotocoagulation (CPC) are presented. The newer laser technique,
selective laser trabeculoplasty, which was shown to be
equally effective as ALT, has the advantage of selectively
targeting pigmented trabecular meshwork cells without
causing coagulation necrosis. Diode lasers with G-probe
are widely used for transscleral photocoagulation of the
ciliary body. Endoscopic CPC has the advantage of directly visualizing treated ciliary processes either via the limbal
or the pars plana approach. Lasers are used for suture lysis
after filtration surgery, opening the occluded tubes of
drainage devices, goniopuncture after a nonpenetrating
deep sclerectomy, and in aqueous misdirection syndrome. From the patient's and physician's perspectives,
laser therapy is less invasive and more easily performed
than most incisional ophthalmic surgeries. In patients
with newly diagnosed and medically uncontrolled glaucoma, 'blebless', safe and successful procedures when repeated would be desirable, and it is possible that lasers
will have an important role in surgical management in the
future.   © 2016 S. Karger AG, Basel

Introduction – Principles of Laser-Tissue Interactions

Clinical use of lasers is based on three basic light-
tissue interactions: photocoagulation, photodisruption, and photoablation. Although there are
exceptions, the wavelength produced by a laser
generally determines which of the three types of
light-tissue interaction will occur. Visible wavelength produces photocoagulation, ultraviolet
yields photoablation, and infrared is used in photodisruption or photocoagulation.

Clinical examples of photocoagulation in
glaucoma therapy include argon laser trabeculoplasty (ALT), peripheral iridotomy, and cyclophotocoagulation (CPC) of ciliary processes.
The types of lasers most frequently used to produce photocoagulation include the argon green
or blue-green laser (514 or 488 nm), the diode
laser (810 nm near infrared), and the frequency-
doubled neodymium-doped yttrium aluminum
garnet (Nd:YAG) laser (532 nm green). Target
and neighboring tissue damage depends on the
duration, spot size, power setting, and pigmentation of the tissue. An increase in exposure time
only modestly increases the lesion's diameter. A
tenfold increase in exposure time roughly dou-

bles lesion diameter and also extends the damage deeper into the target tissue. An increase in power has a strong influence on lesion diameter. Doubling the laser power almost doubles the size of the lesion created. Such increases in laser power create more damage and can be painful to the patient. This can be avoided in some cases by increasing the exposure time rather than laser power.

Control of laser spot size is important in order to achieve the desired therapeutic effect. When broader areas of tissue are treated, a larger spot size such as 200–500 µm (e.g. argon laser iridoplasty) is preferred.

Photodisruption is mainly a mechanical effect. Highly focused laser light produces an optical breakdown with formation of vapor, which quickly collapses and produces a miniature thunderclap. Acoustic shock waves from the thunderclap cause most of the tissue damage. The main example of photodisruption is the peripheral iridotomy produced by the infrared Nd:YAG laser with a wavelength of 1,064 nm.

Photoablation breaks the chemical bonds within the tissue by absorption of photons that hold tissue together without external physical pressure. The laser is able to remove tissue more precisely and with less damage to the surrounding tissue than surgical instruments. Different lasers, such as erbium YAG and femtosecond lasers, have been used for dissecting scleral flaps in deep sclerectomy.

Lasers emit light either continuously or in pulses. A continuous laser modality delivers more overall energy to a target tissue, but it does so over a relatively long time. A pulsed laser produces only modest amounts of energy, but the energy is concentrated into very brief periods, and so each pulse has a relatively high power (power is energy per unit time).

Laser procedures in glaucoma therapy are used to increase aqueous humor outflow, improve or reduce internal block of aqueous humor flow, and to reduce aqueous humor production.

Laser Procedures Increasing Aqueous Humor Outflow

Laser Trabeculoplasty

Laser trabeculoplasty (LT) using an argon laser and the current treatment protocol was first introduced in 1979 [1]. ALT, applied in continuous mode, produces coagulative necrosis and thermal injury to the trabecular meshwork and surrounding tissue. In 1998, pulsed LT using Q-switched frequency-doubled Nd:YAG laser (532 nm) was introduced and the procedure called selective LT (SLT). This laser emits light in short pulses, which are shorter than the thermal relaxation time of the cell (approximately 1 ms) and selectively targets pigmented trabecular meshwork cells without damage to the trabecular meshwork and surrounding tissue [2, 3]. Recently, a micropulse diode laser has been used to perform LT [4–6].

Indication

LT is indicated for lowering of intraocular pressure (IOP) in primary open-angle, exfoliative, and pigmentary glaucoma, as well as high-risk ocular hypertension when IOP is not satisfactorily controlled with medication or as initial treatment.

Mechanism

The mechanism of IOP lowering by LT is not completely understood. The mechanical theory suggests that coagulation necrosis of the trabecular meshwork at the site of laser application causes contraction of trabecular beams. This exerts a pull on the surrounding beams and widens the intertrabecular spaces resulting in lowering of IOP. However, the mechanical mechanism cannot explain similar IOP-lowering efficacy of the SLT that does not produce any thermal damage. Biological mechanisms suggest that increased aqueous outflow results from a number of events, in particular secretion of cytokines, induction of matrix metalloproteinases, increased cell division, repopulation of burn sites, and recruitment of macrophages [7–10].

Table 1. Laser parameters for LT

Laser parameters	ALT	SLT
Spot size	50 µm	400 µm
Exposure	0.1 s	3 ns (fixed)
Power	500–1,200 mW according to the reaction on the TM; with heavily pigmented TM, low power is sufficient	0.4–1.2 mJ according to the desired reaction; in heavily pigmented TM, start with low levels, e.g. 0.4 mJ
Optimal reaction	Transient bleaching or small gas bubble formation	The power is titrated until the appearance of tiny air bubbles ('champagne bubbles') at the site of the laser burn; then, the power is reduced by increments of 0.1 mJ until there are no visible bubbles[1]
Spot number	50–100 evenly spaced spots over 180–360°	50–100 nonoverlapping spots spaced over 180–360°

TM = Trabecular meshwork.

[1] Some continue with the power that causes champagne bubble formation.

Technique

Instillation of a topical α_2-agonist (brimonidine or 1% apraclonidine) to prevent IOP spikes 1 h prior to the procedure and immediately afterwards is advisable. After topical anesthesia, various lenses may be used such as a Goldmann-type gonioscopy, CGA, Ritch trabeculoplasty, or Latina (SLT) lens. After inspecting all quadrants and identifying angle landmarks, the laser burns are placed between the anterior pigmented trabecular meshwork and the nonpigmented trabecular meshwork over 180 or 360°.

Laser parameters for LT are summarized in table 1. In ALT, a spot size of 50 µm, 0.1-second duration, is centered at the junction of pigmented and nonpigmented trabecular meshwork, and the power (500–1,200 mW) titrated to achieve blanching or small gas bubble formation. The power depends on the pigmentation of the trabecular meshwork; with heavily pigmented trabecular meshwork, low power is sufficient. In SLT, a spot size of 400 µm, 3-ns duration (de-pending on the laser type), the power is usually started at 0.8 mJ and titrated until the appearance of tiny air bubbles ('champagne bubbles') at the site of the burn. Then, the power is reduced by increments of 0.1 mJ. Some continue treatment with the power that causes champagne bubble formation. In heavily pigmented trabecular meshwork, treatment is started at low levels, e.g. 0.4 mJ. No blanching is observed with SLT. Laser fluency, defined as laser pulse energy delivered over the spot area, is much smaller for SLT (0.5–1.0 J/cm^2) than ALT (2.0–3.6 × 10^3 J/cm^2).

After LT, instillation of topical anti-inflammatory drops or nonsteroidal drops 3–4 times daily for 5–7 days is optional. It was suggested that anti-inflammatory therapy could modify the clinical effect of SLT mediated by the release of inflammatory mediators that increase the permeability of trabecular meshwork endothelial cells. Recent studies found no influence of anti-inflammatory therapy on the IOP-lowering effect of SLT [11, 12].

Complications

The most common adverse events include elevation of IOP and mild anterior chamber inflammation. An increase in IOP was reported in 0–34% of treated patients depending on the definition of IOP increase and pretreatment with topical hypotensive medications [13–15]. Patients with heavily pigmented trabecular meshwork have a higher risk for IOP elevation after SLT and should be monitored 1–3 h after the procedure [16]. Anterior chamber inflammation is transient and mild [17]. Peripheral anterior synechiae were reported after ALT in 12–47% with higher power and placement of burns to the posterior trabecular meshwork [18, 19]. Recently, formation of peripheral anterior synechiae after repeat SLT were observed [20]. After SLT, dark spots in the corneal endothelium were observed in corneas with pigment on endothelium using specular microscopy. These changes resolved after 1 month [21]. Rare adverse effects published in case reports include: cystoid macular edema, severe anterior uveitis, and subretinal fluid accumulation [22–24].

Efficacy of Selective versus Argon Laser Trabeculoplasty in Medically Treated Patients [17]

In randomized controlled trials, SLT was as effective as ALT in reducing IOP [25]. Most of the trials compared 180° SLT with 180° ALT in patients with medically uncontrolled IOP and found that the mean IOP reduction from baseline ranged from 12 to 28% [26–30]. Success of LT defined as IOP reduction ≥20% was achieved in approximately 60% of the eyes 1 year after LT [29, 31]. In patients with previous 360° ALT, SLT may be more effective as an adjunctive therapy [31, 32].

Efficacy of Laser Trabeculoplasty as Initial Treatment versus Medication

The Glaucoma Laser Trial, including 271 newly diagnosed patients randomized to topical timolol or ALT, found that initial treatment with ALT was at least as efficacious as initial treatment with topical medication after a median follow-up of 7 years [33, 34]. At the time of the Glaucoma Laser Trial, prostaglandin analogs were not available. More recently, SLT has been used as initial treatment in patients with open-angle glaucoma and ocular hypertension, and IOP reduction from baseline was approximately 30% after 180° SLT and was as effective as initial treatment with latanoprost at 12 months [35, 36]. Nagar et al. [15] compared 90, 180, and 360° SLT with latanoprost medical treatment and found no statistical difference in the success rate (>20 and >30% IOP reduction) between 360° SLT and latanoprost. Katz et al. [37] randomized patients for initial treatment to the 360° SLT or the medical arm, and found similar IOP reduction in both arms after 9–12 months of follow-up with more steps necessary to maintain target IOP in the medical arm.

Efficacy of Laser Trabeculoplasty in Different Types of Glaucoma and Secondary Ocular Hypertension

In primary open-angle and exfoliative glaucoma, ALT and SLT as initial and adjunctive treatment have similar good IOP-lowering efficacy [13, 38–41]. Most of the trials were nonrandomized with a short follow-up. Only one nonrandomized prospective trial had a longer follow-up of 30 months including a small number of patients [39].

In normal pressure glaucoma, a single session of 360° SLT achieved 15% reduction from baseline 1 year after laser treatment and reduced the number of medications by 27% [42].

In pseudophakic eyes, ALT and SLT have a similar effect [43]. There was no difference in the success rate (≥20% IOP decrease) after 360° SLT between pseudophakic and phakic eyes at the 12-month follow-up [44].

In pigmentary glaucoma, LT induced a good initial IOP-lowering response, a higher incidence of IOP spikes, and a better chance of success in younger patients [45, 46]. In a retrospective study including 30 patients, the average time to failure after 180° SLT was 27.4 months [47]. Failure was defined if any or more of the following criteria were met: <20% IOP reduction, change in the medical treatment, performance of a further SLT treatment, and referral for surgery.

In primary juvenile open-angle glaucoma and uveitic glaucoma, ALT has a poor response [48, 49]. In the Advanced Glaucoma Intervention Study, risk factors for failure of ALT were younger age and higher IOP [50]. Liu and Birt [26] compared IOP-lowering efficacy of ALT and SLT in a randomized prospective trial including 42 younger medically treated patients who had one eye randomized to ALT or SLT. Mean change from baseline 2 years after laser therapy was 11% for the ALT (22 patients) and 7% for the SLT group (20 patients). Of the 42 patients, only 4 in the ALT and 6 patients in the SLT group had a diagnosis of juvenile open-angle glaucoma, and, due to this small number, subgroup analysis was not performed.

SLT was used to prevent and lower an IOP increase induced by intravitreal injection of triamcinolone acetonide in a small number of patients [51, 52]. The prophylactic use of SLT reduced the need for hypotensive medications in patients with a baseline IOP of 21 mm Hg or more [52].

Predictors of Response to Intraocular Pressure Lowering
With ALT, a lower success rate was reported in eyes without pigmentation of the trabecular meshwork, higher pre-ALT IOP, and in younger patients [50, 53].

For SLT, a higher pre-SLT IOP was associated with a better outcome [54, 55]. Also, a decrease in IOP 2 weeks after SLT to the target IOP predicted low IOP at week 4 and month 3 [56]. Patients' characteristics (age, gender, type of glaucoma medication, and pigmentation of the trabecular meshwork) did not predict the outcome of SLT [55, 57].

Duration of the Effect
The treatment effect of LT diminishes over time. Bovell et al. [32] reported 5-year follow-up data of 152 patients (176 eyes) on maximally tolerated medical treatment randomized to SLT or ALT. Success was defined as ≥20% IOP lowering from baseline with no additional medical, laser, or surgical interventions. Lowering of IOP was similar in the ALT and SLT group over the 5-year period. The success rate was 66% in eyes at 12 months and decreased to 31% at 5 years. Survival analysis indicated that the time to 50% failure in each group is approximately 2 years.

Efficacy and Safety of Repeat Laser Trabeculoplasty
Repeat ALT was successful (defined as IOP <22 mm Hg) in 21–70% of the eyes at 1 year [58, 59]. Long-term success of repeat 360° ALT, defined as a ≥3-mm Hg decrease in IOP to <22 mm Hg without further surgical intervention, was evaluated retrospectively in 44 patients (50 eyes). Repeat ALT was successful in 35% of the eyes at 6 months, 21% at 12 months, 11% at 24 months, and in 5% at 48 months. None of the eyes was successful at 12 months if repeat ALT was performed <12 months after the first ALT [59]. ALT causes thermal damage, inflammatory reactions with activation of fibroblasts, and scar formation. Failure of repeat ALT and an increase in IOP were correlated with the formation of membrane covering the chamber angle [60].

Minimal structural changes to the trabecular meshwork after SLT make this modality potentially repeatable. There is insufficient good quality evidence about the efficacy and safety of repeat SLT. The studies are retrospective chart reviews including a relatively small number of patients with the longest follow-up being 24 months [61–63]. Hong et al. [61] evaluated the efficacy of repeat 360° SLT in 44 eyes (35 patients) with open-angle glaucoma not controlled with maximally tolerable therapy performed at least 6 months after initially successful 360° SLT. Repeat SLT was less efficacious than initial SLT at 1–3 months, with average decreases of –2.9 mm Hg for repeat and –5.0 mm Hg for initial SLT (p = 0.01), but the difference was not significant at 5–8 months. Repeat SLT performed 6–12 months after initial SLT achieved a similar reduction in IOP as repeat SLT performed 12 months or more after initial SLT. In a retrospective study including 42 eyes of 42 patients, Avery et al. [62] demonstrated that repeat SLT had a similar success rate and a longer duration of IOP reduction than primary initial SLT in patients with primary open-angle glaucoma. The success rate (IOP decrease of at least 20% vs. baseline) for first repeat SLT was 66% (mean duration of success of 13 months) and 53% for the second repeat SLT (mean duration of success 9 months). The study has several limitations: for primary initial SLT only 40–50 spots instead of 100 spots were applied over 360°, first repeat SLT was performed as early as 1 month after primary SLT, and only 9 patients had second repeat SLT. Also, follow-up is short: data are shown for 4 weeks and an average of 4 months after the first repeat SLT, and only 28 of 42 patients were followed until failure of the first repeat SLT.

Recently, 360° repeat SLT, including 25 patients (45 eyes) with open-angle glaucoma on medical treatment, was successful (IOP reduction >20%) in 29% of the eyes up to 24 months [63].

Cost-Effectiveness of Laser Trabeculoplasty

Using the Markov model with 25-year horizon, LT may be a more cost-effective treatment option than topical generic prostaglandin analogs when assuming a realistic level of medication adherence in the treatment of newly diagnosed mild open-angle glaucoma (mean deviation of standard automated perimetry <–6 dB) [64]. In Canada, the projected 6-year costs per patient were lower for primary SLT than primary medical treatment for patients aged 65 years or more assuming the following scenarios: a duration of the SLT effect of 2–3 years, when repeated equally effective, and successful in all eyes [65]. Using a simulation model, Cantor et al. [66] compared the total treatment costs of LT versus treatment with medication alone or with filtering surgery in patients with primary open-angle glaucoma not adequately controlled by two medications. Over a 5-year period, LT was associated with the lowest total costs among the treatment strategies.

Summary

LT is a safe procedure and easy to perform, but it is less efficacious in reducing IOP than incisional surgery. Primary LT is as effective as prostaglandin analog monotherapy. It delays the need for topical medication in patients with newly diagnosed open-angle glaucoma and high-risk ocular hypertension. This may reduce side effects of topical medication, and improve adherence and the quality of life. LT is not effective in juvenile open-angle and uveitic glaucoma and, therefore, should not be used. LT may be a more cost-effective option in patients with mild open-angle glaucoma as initial treatment. Compared to ALT, SLT causes minimal structural changes to the trabecular meshwork and is potentially repeatable. However, there are only a few studies including a small number of patients with short follow-ups that support its efficacy and safety when repeated.

Laser Filtration Procedures

Revision of Late-Failing Blebs

Nd:YAG laser was used to improve outflow after trabeculectomy in eyes with episcleral fibrosis [67]. Such failing blebs are often elevated, avascular, and have a double wall on ultrasound biomicroscopy. Using an iridotomy lens (e.g. Abraham lens), the laser was focused on scar tissue within the bleb transconjunctivally and reduced IOP in 24 of 30 patients. The IOP reduction was maintained at 12 months.

Laser Suture Lysis

When not using releasable sutures, an argon laser can be used to cut the sutures and increase the outflow after trabeculectomy. External ligatures around the tubes of nonvalved drainage implants (e.g. Baerveldt) can be cut by an argon laser. After topical instillation of anesthetic drops and optional instillation of 2.5% phenylephrine to reduce the bleeding, a laser beam is applied through a lens (Mandelkorn, Zeiss lens, or similar). The parameters used are: power 300–400 mW, duration 0.1 s, and spot size 50–100 µm, usually 1–3 shots.

Nd:YAG Laser Goniopuncture

Laser goniopuncture is required in approximately 60–70% of eyes with an increase in IOP due to insufficient filtration through a trabeculo-Descemet's membrane after deep sclerectomy. After topical instillation of anesthetic, a gonioscopy lens is used (e.g. GCAL gonioscopy lens, Haag-Streit) to deliver laser energy 2–6 mJ per burst. Usually 1–20 shots are necessary to create a hole in the trabeculo-Descemet's membrane. It is an effective procedure to further lower IOP after deep sclerectomy. IOP <15 mm Hg was achieved and maintained for 2 or more years after single Nd:YAG goniopuncture in about 50% of cases [68]. Failure of laser goniopuncture was associated with iris covering the trabeculo-Descemet's membrane. Complications after laser goniopuncture in 173 eyes included peripheral anterior synechiae in 13%, hypotony in 7%, late acute rise in IOP in 1.7%, blebitis in two eyes, and delayed bleb in one eye [68].

Nd:YAG Laser Photodisruption for Occluded Tubes of Drainage Devices

The laser procedure is performed when lumen of the tube is occluded by iris, inflammatory debris, membrane, or vitreous. Preoperative topical anesthetic is instilled, and an Abraham iridotomy lens is used. If the tube is covered by iris, pretreatment with argon laser (power 250–300 mW, duration 0.1–0.2 s, spot size 500 µm) is followed by Nd:YAG laser (energy 1.0–1.5 mJ/shot). If a lot of vitreous occludes the tube tip, laser treatment should be avoided and a surgical option – vitrectomy – considered [69].

Laser for Sclerostomy and Dissection of Scleral Flaps in Deep Sclerectomy

Ab externo thermal sclerostomies were performed with longer wavelength laser in infrared ranges (holmium:YAG), and ab interno sclerostomies using erbium:YAG laser and endoscopy. Erbium:YAG laser in a pulsed mode was used for dissecting a deep corneoscleral lamella in deep sclerectomy [70]. Other lasers that were tested in animal eyes for dissection of the deep corneoscleral lamella include: CO_2, excimer, and femtosecond laser. Excimer laser has the advantage of dissecting without thermal damage and achieving a smooth tissue surface [71].

Laser Procedures Reducing Internal Block of Aqueous Humor Flow

Laser Peripheral Iridotomy
Indications
It is performed in clinically relevant (e.g. acute angle closure attack) or suspected pupillary block. Laser peripheral iridotomy (LPI) is aimed at preventing acute and chronic angle closure (to prevent the development of peripheral anterior synechiae).

Mechanism
In the pupillary block, the flow of aqueous is impeded from the posterior chamber through the pupil to the anterior chamber. Consequently, the pressure in the posterior chamber increases pushing the peripheral iris forward, which comes into contact with the trabecular meshwork. LPI equalizes the pressure gradient between the anterior and the posterior chamber and opens the chamber angle.

Technique
Topical pilocarpine 2% is instilled to stretch the iris. To prevent postoperative IOP increase, instillation of topical α_2-agonists (apraclonidine 1% or brimonidine) or peroral acetazolamide is given

Table 2. Laser parameters for Nd:YAG laser iridotomy

Power	1–6 mJ
Spot size	50–70 µm (constant for each laser model)
Pulses per burst	1–3
Recommendations	Set defocus to zero Focus the beam within the iris stroma rather than on the surface of the iris[1] Avoid any apparent iris vessels Use the *least amount* of energy that is effective Lens capsule damage is possible >2 mJ of energy With most lasers <5 mJ/pulse is required

[1] Pretreatment with argon laser to minimize bleeding by coagulating iris vessels is optional (spot size 400 µm, duration 0.2 s, energy ~200–300 mW).

prior and immediately after LPI. In acute angle closure attack, topical (e.g. glycerin 10%) or systemic hyperosmotic agents are often necessary to clear corneal edema. After topical anesthesia, an iridotomy lens (e.g. Abraham iridotomy lens) is used. The site of iridotomy is usually placed in the superior quadrants of the iris covered by the upper lid in a thin area or an iris crypt to reduce visual symptoms [72]. Recently, a randomized prospective trial did not find any difference in visual symptoms between participants with totally covered, partially covered, or totally uncovered LPI [73]. Vera et al. [74] observed that temporal LPI placement was less likely to cause linear dysphotopsia than superior placement. The recommended size of LPI is at least 150 µm in diameter to provide an adequate safety margin to account for posttreatment iris edema, pigment epithelial proliferation, or pupil dilation [75]. Usually, Nd:YAG laser is used; pretreatment with argon laser is optional. However, in thick, dark irides, pretreatment with argon reduces total Nd:YAG energy [76]. In tables 2 and 3, laser parameters for Nd:YAG and argon LPI are summarized.

After the procedure, IOP is checked within 1–3 h, and topical corticosteroids are prescribed 2–4 times daily for 4–7 days. Perform gonioscopy regularly to check the angle width and the presence of goniosynechiae. If LPI is patent and the angle does not open, consider other mechanisms of angle closure.

Complications

During the procedure, bleeding from the vessels at the iridotomy site is common and can be easily stopped by gently pressing the contact lens to the eye. Damage to the corneal endothelium may develop especially in eyes with small iris-to-endothelium distance [77]. Postoperative transient elevation in IOP is the most common side effect and occurs 1 h after LPI in approximately 10% of primary angle closure suspect eyes [78]. Visual disturbances (glare, halo, lines, crescent, ghost image, or blurring) occur in 6–12% of the patients [72, 74, 78].

Efficacy of Laser Peripheral Iridotomy in Pigment Dispersion Syndrome

LPI has been proposed to eliminate reverse pupillary block in eyes with pigment dispersion syndrome and decrease dispersion of pigment from the posterior surface of the iris and the consequent IOP increase [79]. In eyes with this syndrome, LPI reduced and delayed the onset of hypertension, especially in eyes that responded with elevation of at least 5 mm Hg after drug-induced

Table 3. Laser parameters for continuous-wave argon laser iridotomy

Medium brown irides	
Preparatory stretch burns	
Spot size, µm	200–500
Exposure time, s	0.2–0.6
Power, mW	200–600
Penetration burns	
Spot size, µm	50
Exposure time, s	0.1–0.2
Power, mW	700–1,500
Average	1,000
Pale blue or hazel irides	
1st step: to obtain a gas bubble	
Spot size, µm	50
Exposure time, s	0.5
Power, mW	1,500
2nd step: penetration through the gas bubble	
Spot size, µm	50
Exposure, s	0.05
Power, mW	1,000
Thick, dark brown irides (chipping technique)	
Spot size, µm	50
Exposure time, s	0.02
Power, mW	1,500

mydriasis [80, 81]. In eyes with increased IOP after dilation, LPI may be considered. However, LPI showed no benefit in preventing progression from pigment dispersion syndrome with ocular hypertension to pigmentary glaucoma within 3 years of follow-up [82].

Laser Iridoplasty
Indications
Indications are appositional angle closure in the presence of patent iridotomy (e.g. iris plateau syndrome) in an eye without peripheral anterior synechiae [83]. The purpose is to enlarge the angle and prevent progressive synechial closure. In acute primary angle closure, laser iridoplasty can be as effective as medications at breaking an acute attack, and it should be considered if an attack cannot be broken by other means [84].

Mechanism
Laser burns applied to the peripheral iris cause its contraction and pull it out of the angle. A fibroblastic membrane is formed and the laser-treated area remains thinner [85].

Technique
Different types of lasers can be used for photocoagulation: argon, diode, and frequency-doubled Nd:YAG lasers. Instillation of pilocarpine to stretch the iris is followed by a topical α_2-agonist prior and after the procedure to prevent IOP elevation. An iridotomy lens is used. Laser parameters vary and depend on the color of the iris (spot size 200–500 µm, duration 0.3–0.5 s, power 200–400 mW). Contraction burns are placed at the most peripheral part of the iris avoiding radial vessels. Optimal reaction is visible contraction and flattening of the iris. A higher power is required for light-colored irides. Postoperative corticosteroids or non-steroidal anti-inflammatory drops are instilled for 4–7 days 3–4 times daily.

Complications
Complications are mild anterior uveitis, corneal endothelial burns, transient elevation in IOP, posterior synechiae, iris atrophy, and a fixed-dilated pupil, which may be permanent [86].

Efficacy
There is no strong evidence for the use of iridoplasty in nonacute angle closure [87]. Only one randomized controlled trial compared the efficacy and safety of LPI with or without laser iridoplasty in Chinese patients with primary angle closure [88]. At the 1-year follow-up, there was no difference in IOP, medication, and need for surgery between the LPI alone and the LPI plus iridoplasty eyes. However, a decrease in peripheral anterior synechiae was noted in the LPI combined with iridoplasty group versus LPI alone, but the sample size was small and indentation gonioscopy was not performed. In a chart review of 14 patients (23 eyes) with iris plateau syndrome, laser iridoplasty

Anesthesia	Retrobulbar or peribulbar injection of a 50:50 mixture of 2% lidocaine and 0.75% bupivacaine with hyaluronidase
G-probe positioning	The G-probe footplate is placed on the conjunctiva with the short side adjacent to the limbus, which positions the fiber-optic tip 1.2 mm behind the limbus; the ciliary body should be identified with transillumination as its position may vary and the placement of the G-probe adjusted accordingly [97]
Scleral transillumination	The fiber-optic light source is directed ~4 mm posterior to the corneoscleral limbus to identify the ciliary body by transillumination; the dark demarcation line indicates the anterior margin of the ciliary body
Settings	Recommended setting: duration of 2 s, from 1,500 mW for dark- to 2,000 mW for light-colored irides, and increase the energy until an audible 'pop' is heard indicating tissue disruption; if a 'pop' sound occurs during two sequential subsequent laser applications, the power is reduced by 150 mW and treatment completed at this power [98]
Applications	10–20 over 180°, energy 5–6 J/pulse, total treatment per session up to 270° of circumference avoiding 3- and 9-o'clock positions (to avoid long posterior ciliary nerves); some surgeons prefer to use low energy and more applications; retreatments are often needed, but the incidence of severe complications is low

was long-term effective in eliminating residual angle closure after LPI [89]. In Chinese patients with acute primary angle closure, argon laser iridoplasty was safe and significantly more reduced IOP within the first 2 h than conventional systemic medications [90]. At the 15-month follow-up, there was no difference in mean IOP and requirement for glaucoma drugs between acute primary angle closure eyes treated with laser iridoplasty and systemic medications [91].

Laser Procedures Reducing Aqueous Humor Production

Cyclophotocoagulation
Indications
CPC is indicated to lower IOP in glaucoma that is refractory to medical or surgical treatment, where previous filtration surgery has failed or is likely to fail, as an alternative to drainage devices, or after previous failure of a glaucoma drainage device. Transscleral CPC may be successful in the medi-cally uncontrolled and refractory aqueous misdirection syndrome [92, 93].

Laser Types
Lasers most frequently used in the continuous mode for CPC are diode and argon lasers. Laser treatment is delivered as transscleral or endoscopic approach, rarely as transpupilar approach in cases of aniridia or broad iridectomy. Recently, transscleral diode laser CPC in micropulse mode has been introduced [94].

Ultrasound cyclocoagulation using high-intensity focused ultrasound delivered by a circular miniaturized device containing six piezoceramic transducers has been used to destroy ciliary processes [95].

Mechanism
Diode laser CPC causes thermal damage to ciliary processes with a reduction in aqueous humor production [96]. With increasing time following treatment, ciliary epithelium proliferates and this may account for late treatment failure. In the

aqueous misdirection syndrome, it is assumed that coagulative necrosis and shrinkage of ciliary processes disrupts the ciliary-hyaloid interface. The decreased aqueous formation and posterior rotation of ciliary processes may reestablish the normal aqueous flow from the posterior to the anterior chamber.

Technique
Transscleral CPC with diode laser using G-probe is the procedure of choice, because of its low incidence of complications compared with other cyclodestructive procedures. The technique for CPC with diode laser and G-probe is summarized in table 4.

In endoscopic CPC, a 20-gauge fiber-optic cable connected to the laser unit delivers diode laser energy to the ciliary processes which are visualized during treatment [99]. The optimal reaction is whitening and shrinkage of ciliary processes. The probe is introduced either pars plana and combined with vitrectomy or a limbal approach is used as stand-alone procedure or combined with cataract surgery, treating 270–300°. In mild-to-moderate open-angle medically controlled glaucoma, compared to cataract surgery alone, endoscopic CPC combined with cataract extraction reduced the number of glaucoma medications and may delay glaucoma progression in patients with mild-to-moderate glaucoma [100, 101].

Postoperative topical cycloplegic agents and corticosteroids are instilled 3–4 times daily for 2–3 weeks. Topical and systemic antiglaucoma medications are titrated according to the IOP. Effectiveness of CPC is assessed after 4 weeks.

Complications
Complications include uveitis, IOP spikes, hyphema, cataract progression, vitreous hemorrhage, malignant glaucoma, vison loss, persistent hypotony, and phthisis. Serious complications are higher following high treatment energy per session and in neovascular and uveitic glaucoma [102, 103]. The complications reported with high-intensity focused ultrasound cyclocoagulation included conjunctival hyperemia, superficial keratitis, anterior chamber inflammation, and corneal edema [104].

Efficacy
The effect of transscleral diode CPC among studies is difficult to compare, because of different criteria of success and different patient populations. Reduction in IOP <22 mm Hg was achieved in 54–92.7% of the eyes [103]. Preservation of visual acuity depends mainly on the underlying disease. Some studies found a correlation between the energy delivered and treatment success, whereas others did not find any correlation. Retreatments are necessary in 20–67%. CPC is less effective in pediatric glaucoma and younger patients than in older patients. Recently, in a randomized study including 48 patients with refractory glaucoma, diode transscleral CPC in micropulse mode was equally effective in lowering IOP as transscleral CPC in continuous mode [105]. The micropulse mode provided a more consistent and predictable effect in lowering IOP with minimal ocular complications.

In a prospective study, endoscopic CPC compared to the Ahmed drainage implant achieved similar success (6 mm Hg ≤ IOP ≤ 21 mm Hg) in 68 patients with uncontrolled glaucoma at 2 years. The success was 71% for the Ahmed valve group and 74% for the endoscopic CPC.

Efficacy of high-intensity focused ultrasound cyclocoagulation in medically uncontrolled glaucoma patients (mainly with primary open-angle glaucoma) was evaluated at 12 months. The success (>20% IOP decrease) was achieved in 57% (12/21) in the group with a 4-second duration of each ultrasound shot and in 48% (12/25) in the group with a 6-second duration of each ultrasound shot.

References

1 Wise JB, Witter SL: Argon laser therapy for open-angle glaucoma. A pilot study. Arch Ophthalmol 1979;97:319–322.

2 Kramer TR, Noecker RJ: Comparison of the morphologic changes after selective laser trabeculoplasty and argon laser trabeculoplasty in human eye bank eyes. Ophthalmology 2001;108:773–779.

3 Cvenkel B, Hvala A, Drnovsek-Olup B, Gale N: Acute ultrastructural changes of the trabecular meshwork after selective laser trabeculoplasty and low power argon laser trabeculoplasty. Lasers Surg Med 2003;33:204–208.

4 Detry-Morel M, Muschart F, Pourjavan S: Micropulse diode laser (810 nm) versus argon laser trabeculoplasty in the treatment of open-angle glaucoma: comparative short-term safety and efficacy profile. Bull Soc Belge Ophtalmol 2008;308:21–28.

5 Fea AM, Bosone A, Rolle T, Brogliatti B, Grignolo FM: Micropulse diode laser trabeculoplasty (MDLT): a phase II clinical study with 12 months follow-up. Clin Ophthalmol 2008;2:247–252.

6 Rantala E, Valimaki J: Micropulse diode laser trabeculoplasty – 180-degree treatment. Acta Ophthalmol 2012;90:441–444.

7 Kagan DB, Gorfinkel NS, Hutnik CM: Mechanisms of selective laser trabeculoplasty: a review. Clin Experiment Ophthalmol 2014;42:675–681.

8 Alvarado JA, Katz LJ, Trivedi S, Shifera AS: Monocyte modulation of aqueous outflow and recruitment to the trabecular meshwork following selective laser trabeculoplasty. Arch Ophthalmol 2010;128:731–737.

9 Amelinckx A, Castello M, Arrieta-Quintero E, Lee T, Salas N, Hernandez E, Lee RK, Bhattacharya SK, Parel JM: Laser trabeculoplasty induces changes in the trabecular meshwork glycoproteome: a pilot study. J Proteome Res 2009;8:3727–3736.

10 Izzotti A, Longobardi M, Cartiglia C, Rathschuler F, Sacca SC: Trabecular meshwork gene expression after selective laser trabeculoplasty. PLoS One 2011;6:e20110.

11 Jinapriya D, D'Souza M, Hollands H, El-Defrawy SR, Irrcher I, Smallman D, Farmer JP, Cheung J, Urton T, Day A, Sun X, Campbell RJ: Anti-inflammatory therapy after selective laser trabeculoplasty: a randomized, double-masked, placebo-controlled clinical trial. Ophthalmology 2014;121:2356–2361.

12 Champagne S, Anctil JL, Goyette A, Lajoie C, Des Marchais B: Influence on intraocular pressure of anti-inflammatory treatments after selective laser trabeculoplasty. J Fr Ophtalmol 2015;38:588–594.

13 Kent SS, Hutnik CM, Birt CM, Damji KF, Harasymowycz P, Si F, Hodge W, Pan I, Crichton A: A randomized clinical trial of selective laser trabeculoplasty versus argon laser trabeculoplasty in patients with pseudoexfoliation. J Glaucoma 2015;24:344–347.

14 The Glaucoma Laser Trial. I. Acute effects of argon laser trabeculoplasty on intraocular pressure. Glaucoma Laser Trial Research Group. Arch Ophthalmol 1989;107:1135–1142.

15 Nagar M, Ogunyomade A, O'Brart DP, Howes F, Marshall J: A randomised, prospective study comparing selective laser trabeculoplasty with latanoprost for the control of intraocular pressure in ocular hypertension and open angle glaucoma. Br J Ophthalmol 2005;89:1413–1417.

16 Harasymowycz PJ, Papamatheakis DG, Latina M, De Leon M, Lesk MR, Damji KF: Selective laser trabeculoplasty (SLT) complicated by intraocular pressure elevation in eyes with heavily pigmented trabecular meshworks. Am J Ophthalmol 2005;139:1110–1113.

17 Wong MO, Lee JW, Choy BN, Chan JC, Lai JS: Systematic review and meta-analysis on the efficacy of selective laser trabeculoplasty in open-angle glaucoma. Surv Ophthalmol 2015;60:36–50.

18 Traverso CE, Greenidge KC, Spaeth GL: Formation of peripheral anterior synechiae following argon laser trabeculoplasty. A prospective study to determine relationship to position of laser burns. Arch Ophthalmol 1984;102:861–863.

19 Koller T, Sturmer J, Reme C, Gloor B: Risk factors for development of argon laser trabeculoplasty failure producing membrane in the chamber angle (in German). Ophthalmologe 1996;93:552–557.

20 Baser EF, Akbulut D: Significant peripheral anterior synechiae after repeat selective laser trabeculoplasty. Can J Ophthalmol 2015;50:e36–e38.

21 Ong K, Ong L, Ong L: Corneal endothelial changes after selective laser trabeculoplasty. Clin Experiment Ophthalmol 2013;41:537–540.

22 Ha JH, Bowling B, Chen SD: Cystoid macular oedema following selective laser trabeculoplasty in a diabetic patient. Clin Experiment Ophthalmol 2014;42:200–201.

23 Koktekir BE, Gedik S, Bakbak B: Bilateral severe anterior uveitis after unilateral selective laser trabeculoplasty. Clin Experiment Ophthalmol 2013;41:305–307.

24 Phillis CA, Bourke RD: Bilateral subretinal fluid mimicking subretinal neovascularization within 24 hours after selective laser trabeculoplasty. J Glaucoma 2015;25:e110–e114.

25 McAlinden C: Selective laser trabeculoplasty (SLT) vs other treatment modalities for glaucoma: systematic review. Eye (Lond) 2014;28:249–258.

26 Liu Y, Birt CM: Argon versus selective laser trabeculoplasty in younger patients: 2-year results. J Glaucoma 2012;21:112–115.

27 Damji KF, Shah KC, Rock WJ, Bains HS, Hodge WG: Selective laser trabeculoplasty v argon laser trabeculoplasty: a prospective randomised clinical trial. Br J Ophthalmol 1999;83:718–722.

28 Martinez-de-la-Casa JM, Garcia-Feijoo J, Castillo A, Matilla M, Macias JM, Benitez-del-Castillo JM, Garcia-Sanchez J: Selective vs argon laser trabeculoplasty: hypotensive efficacy, anterior chamber inflammation, and postoperative pain. Eye (Lond) 2004;18:498–502.

29 Damji KF, Bovell AM, Hodge WG, Rock W, Shah K, Buhrmann R, Pan YI: Selective laser trabeculoplasty versus argon laser trabeculoplasty: results from a 1-year randomised clinical trial. Br J Ophthalmol 2006;90:1490–1494.

30 Cvenkel B: One-year follow-up of selective laser trabeculoplasty in open-angle glaucoma. Ophthalmologica 2004;218:20–25.

31 Birt CM: Selective laser trabeculoplasty retreatment after prior argon laser trabeculoplasty: 1-year results. Can J Ophthalmol 2007;42:715–719.

32 Bovell AM, Damji KF, Hodge WG, Rock WJ, Buhrmann RR, Pan YI: Long term effects on the lowering of intraocular pressure: selective laser or argon laser trabeculoplasty? Can J Ophthalmol 2011;46:408–413.

33 The Glaucoma Laser Trial (GLT). 2. Results of argon laser trabeculoplasty versus topical medicines. The Glaucoma Laser Trial Research Group. Ophthalmology 1990;97:1403–1413.

34 The Glaucoma Laser Trial (GLT) and glaucoma laser trial follow-up study: 7. Results. Glaucoma Laser Trial Research Group. Am J Ophthalmol 1995;120:718–731.

35 McIlraith I, Strasfeld M, Colev G, Hutnik CM: Selective laser trabeculoplasty as initial and adjunctive treatment for open-angle glaucoma. J Glaucoma 2006;15:124–130.

36 Melamed S, Ben Simon GJ, Levkovitch-Verbin H: Selective laser trabeculoplasty as primary treatment for open-angle glaucoma: a prospective, nonrandomized pilot study. Arch Ophthalmol 2003;121:957–960.

37 Katz LJ, Steinmann WC, Kabir A, Molineaux J, Wizov SS, Marcellino G, SLT/Med Study Group: Selective laser trabeculoplasty versus medical therapy as initial treatment of glaucoma: a prospective, randomized trial. J Glaucoma 2012;21:460–468.

38 Gracner T: Intraocular pressure response of capsular glaucoma and primary open-angle glaucoma to selective Nd:YAG laser trabeculoplasty: a prospective, comparative clinical trial. Eur J Ophthalmol 2002;12:287–292.

39 Shazly TA, Smith J, Latina MA: Long-term safety and efficacy of selective laser trabeculoplasty as primary therapy for the treatment of pseudoexfoliation glaucoma compared with primary open-angle glaucoma. Clin Ophthalmol 2010;5:5–10.

40 Goldenfeld M, Geyer O, Segev E, Kaplan-Messas A, Melamed S: Selective laser trabeculoplasty in uncontrolled pseudoexfoliation glaucoma. Ophthalmic Surg Lasers Imaging 2011;42:390–393.

41 Ayala M, Chen E: Comparison of selective laser trabeculoplasty (SLT) in primary open angle glaucoma and pseudoexfoliation glaucoma. Clin Ophthalmol 2011;5:1469–1473.

42 Kent SS, Hutnik CM, Birt CM, Damji KF, Harasymowycz P, Si F, Hodge W, Pan I, Crichton A: A randomized clinical trial of selective laser trabeculoplasty versus argon laser trabeculoplasty in patients with pseudoexfoliation. J Glaucoma 2015;24:344–347.

43 Rosenfeld E, Shemesh G, Kurtz S: The efficacy of selective laser trabeculoplasty versus argon laser trabeculoplasty in pseudophakic glaucoma patients. Clin Ophthalmol 2012;6:1935–1940.

44 Seymenoglu G, Baser EF: Efficacy of selective laser trabeculoplasty in phakic and pseudophakic eyes. J Glaucoma 2015;24:105–110.

45 Ritch R, Liebmann J, Robin A, Pollack IP, Harrison R, Levene RZ, Hagadus J: Argon laser trabeculoplasty in pigmentary glaucoma. Ophthalmology 1993;100:909–913.

46 Lunde MW: Argon laser trabeculoplasty in pigmentary dispersion syndrome with glaucoma. Am J Ophthalmol 1983;96:721–725.

47 Ayala M: Long-term outcomes of selective laser trabeculoplasty (SLT) treatment in pigmentary glaucoma patients. J Glaucoma 2014;23:616–619.

48 Horns DJ, Bellows AR, Hutchinson BT, Allen RC: Argon laser trabeculoplasty for open angle glaucoma. A retrospective study of 380 eyes. Trans Ophthalmol Soc UK 1983;103(pt 3):288–296.

49 Robin AL, Pollack IP: Argon laser trabeculoplasty in secondary forms of open-angle glaucoma. Arch Ophthalmol 1983;101:382–384.

50 Fink AI, Jordan AJ, Lao PN, Fong DA: Therapeutic limitations of argon laser trabeculoplasty. Br J Ophthalmol 1988;72:263–269.

51 Rubin B, Taglienti A, Rothman RF, Marcus CH, Serle JB: The effect of selective laser trabeculoplasty on intraocular pressure in patients with intravitreal steroid-induced elevated intraocular pressure. J Glaucoma 2008;17:287–292.

52 Bozkurt E, Kara N, Yazici AT, Yuksel K, Demirok A, Yilmaz OF, Demir S: Prophylactic selective laser trabeculoplasty in the prevention of intraocular pressure elevation after intravitreal triamcinolone acetonide injection. Am J Ophthalmol 2011;152:976–981.e2.

53 Odberg T, Sandvik L: The medium and long-term efficacy of primary argon laser trabeculoplasty in avoiding topical medication in open angle glaucoma. Acta Ophthalmol Scand 1999;77:176–181.

54 Tzimis V, Tze L, Ganesh J, Muhsen S, Kiss A, Kranemann C, Birt CM: Laser trabeculoplasty: an investigation into factors that might influence outcomes. Can J Ophthalmol 2011;46:305–309.

55 Martow E, Hutnik CM, Mao A: SLT and adjunctive medical therapy: a prediction rule analysis. J Glaucoma 2011;20:266–270.

56 Johnson PB, Katz LJ, Rhee DJ: Selective laser trabeculoplasty: predictive value of early intraocular pressure measurements for success at 3 months. Br J Ophthalmol 2006;90:741–743.

57 Singh D, Coote MA, O'Hare F, Walland MJ, Ghosh S, Xie J, Ruddle JB, Crowston JG: Topical prostaglandin analogues do not affect selective laser trabeculoplasty outcomes. Eye (Lond) 2009;23:2194–2199.

58 Weber PA, Burton GD, Epitropoulos AT: Laser trabeculoplasty retreatment. Ophthalmic Surg 1989;20:702–706.

59 Feldman RM, Katz LJ, Spaeth GL, Crapotta JA, Fahmy IA, Ali MA: Long-term efficacy of repeat argon laser trabeculoplasty. Ophthalmology 1991;98:1061–1065.

60 Koller T, Sturmer J, Reme C, Gloor B: Membrane formation in the chamber angle after failure of argon laser trabeculoplasty: analysis of risk factors. Br J Ophthalmol 2000;84:48–53.

61 Hong BK, Winer JC, Martone JF, Wand M, Altman B, Shields B: Repeat selective laser trabeculoplasty. J Glaucoma 2009;18:180–183.

62 Avery N, Ang GS, Nicholas S, Wells A: Repeatability of primary selective laser trabeculoplasty in patients with primary open-angle glaucoma. Int Ophthalmol 2013;33:501–506.

63 Khouri AS, Lari HB, Berezina TL, Maltzman B, Fechtner RD: Long term efficacy of repeat selective laser trabeculoplasty. J Ophthalmic Vis Res 2014;9:444–448.

64 Stein JD, Kim DD, Peck WW, Giannetti SM, Hutton DW: Cost-effectiveness of medications compared with laser trabeculoplasty in patients with newly diagnosed open-angle glaucoma. Arch Ophthalmol 2012;130:497–505.

65 Lee R, Hutnik CM: Projected cost comparison of selective laser trabeculoplasty versus glaucoma medication in the Ontario Health Insurance Plan. Can J Ophthalmol 2006;41:449–456.

66 Cantor LB, Katz LJ, Cheng JW, Chen E, Tong KB, Peabody JW: Economic evaluation of medication, laser trabeculoplasty and filtering surgeries in treating patients with glaucoma in the US. Curr Med Res Opin 2008;24:2905–2918.

67 Weber PA, Jones JH, Kapetansky F: Neodymium: YAG transconjunctival laser revision of late-failing filtering blebs. Ophthalmology 1999;106:2023–2026.

68 Anand N, Pilling R: Nd:YAG laser goniopuncture after deep sclerectomy: outcomes. Acta Ophthalmol 2010;88:110–115.

69 Desatnik HR, Foster RE, Rockwood EJ, Baerveldt G, Meyers SM, Lewis H: Management of glaucoma implants occluded by vitreous incarceration. J Glaucoma 2000;9:311–316.

70 Klink T, Schlunck G, Lieb WE, Klink J, Grehn F: Long-term results of erbium YAG-laser-assisted deep sclerectomy. Eye (Lond) 2008;22:370–374.

71 Klink T, Schlunck G, Lieb W, Klink J, Grehn F: CO_2, excimer and erbium:YAG laser in deep sclerectomy. Ophthalmologica 2008;222:74–80.

72 Spaeth GL, Idowu O, Seligsohn A, Henderer J, Fonatanarosa J, Modi A, Nallamshetty HS, Chieh J, Haim L, Steinmann WC, Moster M: The effects of iridotomy size and position on symptoms following laser peripheral iridotomy. J Glaucoma 2005;14:364–367.

73 Congdon N, Yan X, Friedman DS, Foster PJ, van den Berg TJ, Peng M, Gangwani R, He M: Visual symptoms and retinal straylight after laser peripheral iridotomy: the Zhongshan Angle-Closure Prevention Trial. Ophthalmology 2012;119:1375–1382.

74 Vera V, Naqi A, Belovay GW, Varma DK, Ahmed II: Dysphotopsia after temporal versus superior laser peripheral iridotomy: a prospective randomized paired eye trial. Am J Ophthalmol 2014;157:929–935.

75 Day AC, Foster PJ: How large should an iridotomy be? Br J Ophthalmol 2011;95:747–748.

76 de Silva DJ, Day AC, Bunce C, Gazzard G, Foster PJ: Randomised trial of sequential pretreatment for Nd:YAG laser iridotomy in dark irides. Br J Ophthalmol 2012;96:263–266.

77 Wang PX, Koh VT, Loon SC: Laser iridotomy and the corneal endothelium: a systemic review. Acta Ophthalmol 2014;92:604–616.

78 Jiang Y, Chang DS, Foster PJ, He M, Huang S, Aung T, Friedman DS: Immediate changes in intraocular pressure after laser peripheral iridotomy in primary angle-closure suspects. Ophthalmology 2012;119:283–288.

79 Karickhoff JR: Pigmentary dispersion syndrome and pigmentary glaucoma: a new mechanism concept, a new treatment, and a new technique. Ophthalmic Surg 1992;23:269–277.

80 Gandolfi SA, Vecchi M: Effect of a YAG laser iridotomy on intraocular pressure in pigment dispersion syndrome. Ophthalmology 1996;103:1693–1695.

81 Gandolfi SA, Ungaro N, Tardini MG, Ghirardini S, Carta A, Mora P: A 10-year follow-up to determine the effect of YAG laser iridotomy on the natural history of pigment dispersion syndrome: a randomized clinical trial. JAMA Ophthalmol 2014;132:1433–1438.

82 Scott A, Kotecha A, Bunce C, Balidis M, Garway-Heath DF, Miller MH, Wormald R: YAG laser peripheral iridotomy for the prevention of pigment dispersion glaucoma: a prospective, randomized, controlled trial. Ophthalmology 2011;118:468–473.

83 Ritch R, Tham CC, Lam DS: Argon laser peripheral iridoplasty (ALPI): an update. Surv Ophthalmol 2007;52:279–288.

84 Lai JS, Tham CC, Chua JK, Poon AS, Lam DS: Laser peripheral iridoplasty as initial treatment of acute attack of primary angle-closure: a long-term follow-up study. J Glaucoma 2002;11:484–487.

85 Liu J, Lamba T, Belyea DA: Peripheral laser iridoplasty opens angle in plateau iris by thinning the cross-sectional tissues. Clin Ophthalmol 2013;7:1895–1897.

86 Espana EM, Ioannidis A, Tello C, Liebmann JM, Foster P, Ritch R: Urrets-Zavalia syndrome as a complication of argon laser peripheral iridoplasty. Br J Ophthalmol 2007;91:427–429.

87 Ng WS, Ang GS, Azuara-Blanco A: Laser peripheral iridoplasty for angle-closure. Cochrane Database Syst Rev 2012;2:CD006746.

88 Sun X, Liang YB, Wang NL, Fan SJ, Sun LP, Li SZ, Liu WR: Laser peripheral iridotomy with and without iridoplasty for primary angle-closure glaucoma: 1-year results of a randomized pilot study. Am J Ophthalmol 2010;150:68–73.

89 Ritch R, Tham CC, Lam DS: Long-term success of argon laser peripheral iridoplasty in the management of plateau iris syndrome. Ophthalmology 2004;111:104–108.

90 Lam DS, Lai JS, Tham CC, Chua JK, Poon AS: Argon laser peripheral iridoplasty versus conventional systemic medical therapy in treatment of acute primary angle-closure glaucoma: a prospective, randomized, controlled trial. Ophthalmology 2002;109:1591–1596.

91 Lai JS, Tham CC, Chua JK, Poon AS, Chan JC, Lam SW, Lam DS: To compare argon laser peripheral iridoplasty (ALPI) against systemic medications in treatment of acute primary angle-closure: mid-term results. Eye 2006;20:309–314.

92 Stumpf TH, Austin M, Bloom PA, McNaught A, Morgan JE: Transscleral cyclodiode laser photocoagulation in the treatment of aqueous misdirection syndrome. Ophthalmology 2008;115:2058–2061.

93 Dave P, Senthil S, Rao HL, Garudadri CS: Treatment outcomes in malignant glaucoma. Ophthalmology 2013;120:984–990.

94 Meyer JJ, Lawrence SD: What's new in laser treatment for glaucoma? Curr Opin Ophthalmol 2012;23:111–117.

95 Aptel F, Charrel T, Lafon C, Romano F, Chapelon JY, Blumen-Ohana E, Nordmann JP, Denis P: Miniaturized high-intensity focused ultrasound device in patients with glaucoma: a clinical pilot study. Invest Ophthalmol Vis Sci 2011;52:8747–8753.

96 McKelvie PA, Walland MJ: Pathology of cyclodiode laser: a series of nine enucleated eyes. Br J Ophthalmol 2002;86:381–386.

97 Agrawal P, Martin KR: Ciliary body position variability in glaucoma patients assessed by scleral transillumination. Eye 2008;22:1499–1503.

98 Kosoko O, Gaasterland DE, Pollack IP, Enger CL: Long-term outcome of initial ciliary ablation with contact diode laser transscleral cyclophotocoagulation for severe glaucoma. The Diode Laser Ciliary Ablation Study Group. Ophthalmology 1996;103:1294–1302.

99   Lin S: Endoscopic cyclophotocoagulation. Br J Ophthalmol 2002;86:1434–1438.

100 Francis BA, Berke SJ, Dustin L, Noecker R: Endoscopic cyclophotocoagulation combined with phacoemulsification versus phacoemulsification alone in medically controlled glaucoma. J Cataract Refract Surg 2014;40:1313–1321.

101 Siegel MJ, Boling WS, Faridi OS, Gupta CK, Kim C, Boling RC, Citron ME, Siegel MJ, Siegel LI: Combined endoscopic cyclophotocoagulation and phacoemulsification versus phacoemulsification alone in the treatment of mild to moderate glaucoma. Clin Experiment Ophthalmol 2015;43:531–539.

102 Ramli N, Htoon HM, Ho CL, Aung T, Perera S: Risk factors for hypotony after transscleral diode cyclophotocoagulation. J Glaucoma 2012;21:169–173.

103 Ishida K: Update on results and complications of cyclophotocoagulation. Curr Opin Ophthalmol 2013;24:102–110.

104 Denis P, Aptel F, Rouland JF, Nordmann JP, Lachkar Y, Renard JP, Sellem E, Baudouin C, Bron A: Cyclocoagulation of the ciliary bodies by high-intensity focused ultrasound: a 12-month multicenter study. Invest Ophthalmol Vis Sci 2015;56:1089–1096.

105 Aquino MC, Barton K, Tan AM, Sng C, Li X, Loon SC, Chew PT: Micropulse versus continuous wave transscleral diode cyclophotocoagulation in refractory glaucoma: a randomized exploratory study. Clin Experiment Ophthalmol 2015;43:40–46.

Barbara Cvenkel
Department of Ophthalmology, University Medical Center Ljubljana
Grablovičeva 46
SI–1000 Ljubljana (Slovenia)
E-Mail barbara.cvenkel@gmail.com

Traverso CE, Stalmans I, Topouzis F, Bagnasco L (eds): Glaucoma.
ESASO Course Series. Basel, Karger, 2016, vol 8, pp 91–96 (DOI: 10.1159/000446146)

Canaloplasty

Paolo Brusini

Glaucoma Unit, Città di Udine Health Center, Udine, Italy

Abstract

Canaloplasty is a new nonperforating surgical technique
for open-angle glaucoma, in which a microcatheter is inserted within Schlemm's canal for the entire 360°. A 10-0
prolene suture, which is tied to the distal tip of the microcatheter, is then positioned and left tensioned in
Schlemm's canal, thus facilitating aqueous outflow
through natural pathways. A small amount of viscoelastic agent is delivered to Schlemm's canal while the catheter is withdrawn. The mid-term results are very promising without any signs of serious permanent complications. The most frequent complications observed included hyphema, Descemet's membrane detachment, IOP
spikes, and hypotony. The advantages of canaloplasty
over trabeculectomy include (1) no subconjunctival
bleb, (2) no need for antimetabolites, (3) fewer postoperative complications, and (4) a simplified follow-up. The
disadvantages include (1) a long and rather steep surgical learning curve, (2) the need of specific instruments,
(3) average postoperative intraocular pressure levels
tend not to be very low, and (4) impossibility to perform
the entire procedure in some cases.

Trabeculectomy was first introduced about 50
years ago [1, 2], and, to this day, it is still considered as the gold standard surgical procedure in
glaucoma. This technique is effective and simple
to perform; however, several early and late potentially serious complications can occur, such as
athalamia, hypotonus, choroidal detachment, or
bleb infection. Most of the postoperative complications are related to the subconjunctival bleb. A
number of nonperforating surgical techniques
have been proposed in the past to address the disadvantages of trabeculectomy [3–5]. These surgical options tend to offer lower complication rates,
and postoperative outcomes are less influenced
by conditions of the conjunctiva. Canaloplasty is
a relatively new nonperforating bleb-independent technique derived from Stegmann's viscocanalostomy, in which a 10-0 prolene suture is positioned and tensioned within Schlemm's canal,
thus facilitating aqueous outflow through natural
pathways.

The surgical technique is well known and has
extensively been reported in the literature [6–11].
In brief, surgery starts with a fornix-based conjunctival flap, and a 4 × 4 mm superficial scleral

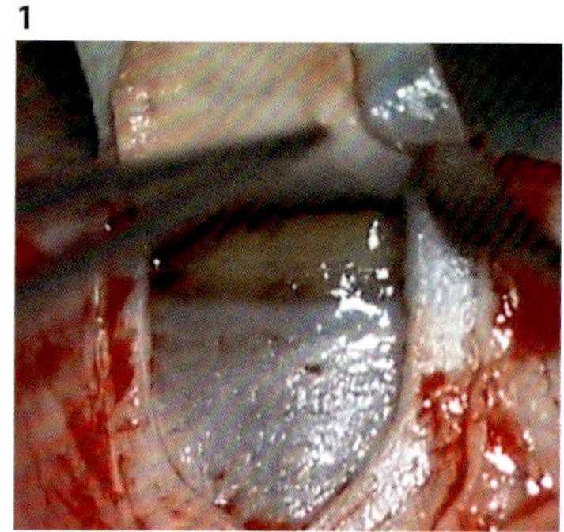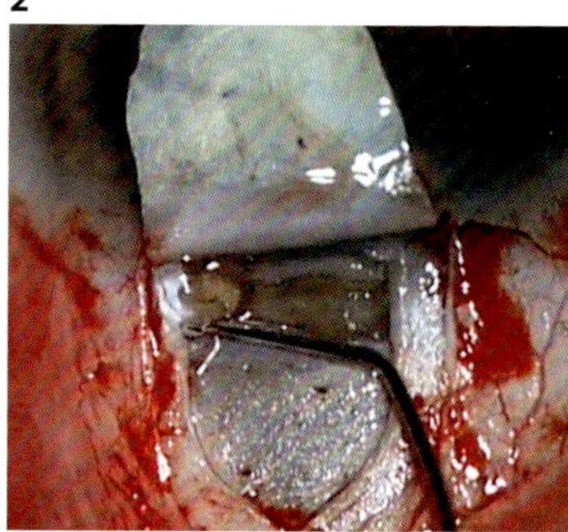

Fig. 1. Deep scleral flap dissection.
Fig. 2. Dilation of Schlemm's canal.

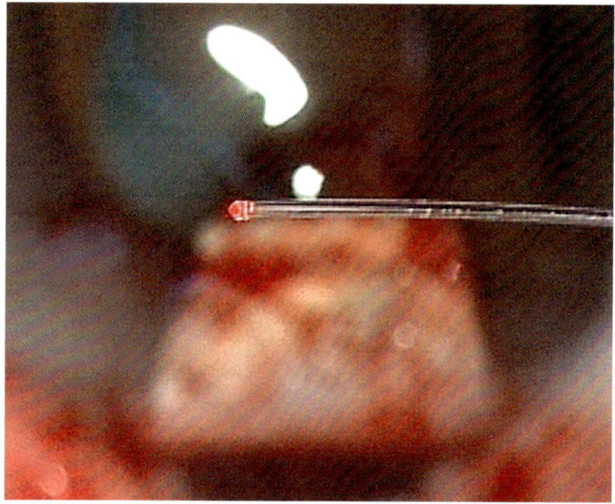

Fig. 3. Lighted final tip of a microcatheter.

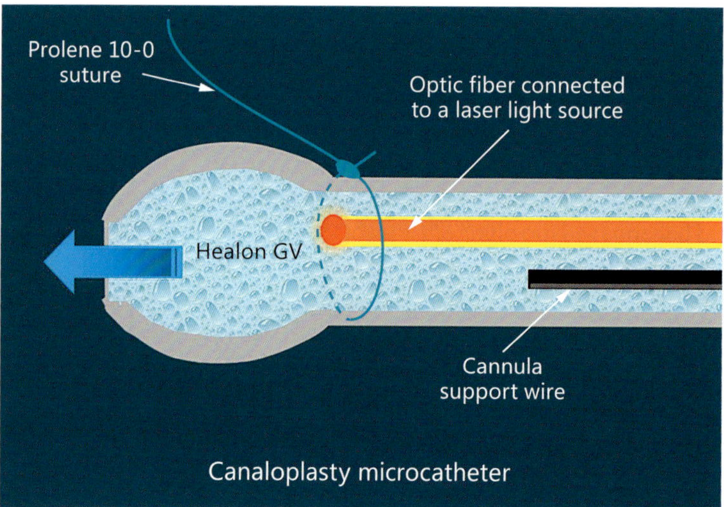

Fig. 4. Schematic view of the microcatheter.

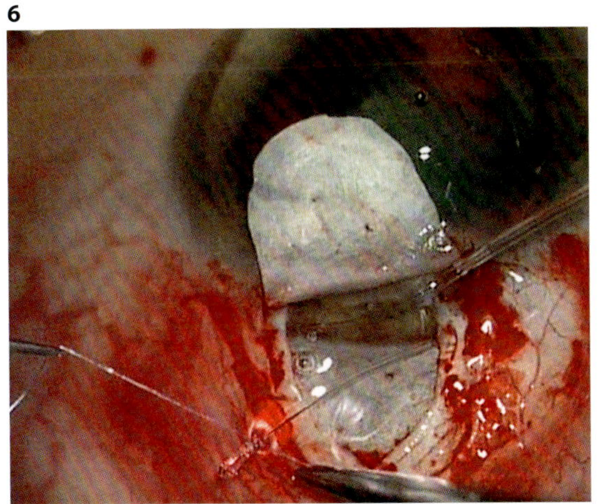

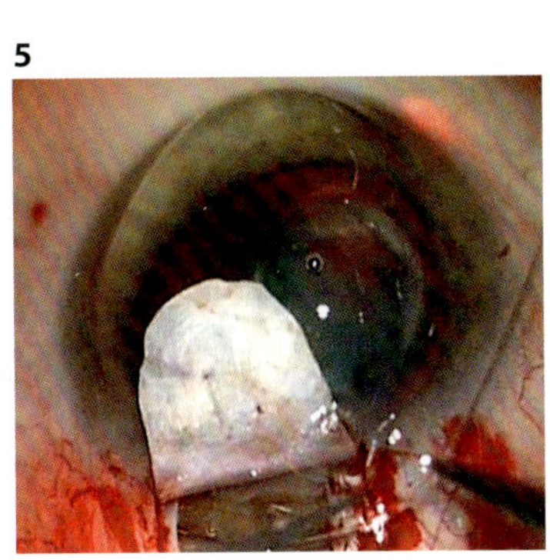

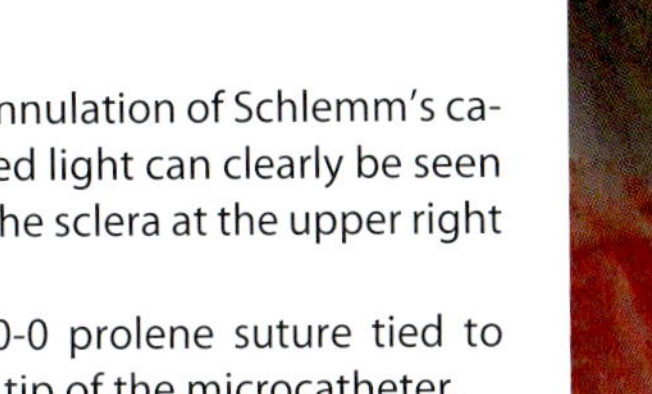

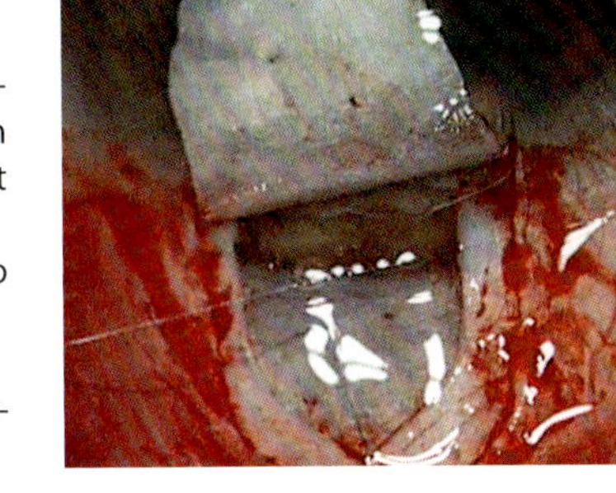

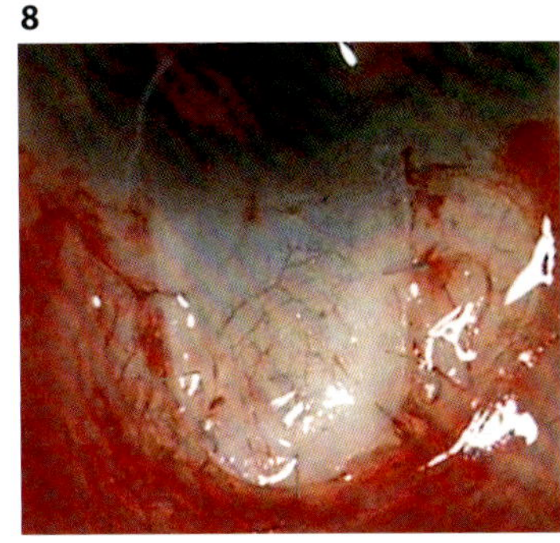

Fig. 5. Cannulation of Schlemm's canal. The red light can clearly be seen through the sclera at the upper right corner.
Fig. 6. 10-0 prolene suture tied to the distal tip of the microcatheter.
Fig. 7. Prolene suture tensioning.
Fig. 8. Suture of the superficial scleral flap.

flap, which is dissected forward into the clear cornea for 1.5 mm. A deep scleral flap is then created, which opens into Schlemm's canal (fig. 1). The deep scleral flap is removed and the two ostia of the canal are dilated and filled with high-molecular-weight hyaluronic acid (fig. 2). A 200-μm microcatheter (iTrack; iScience Interventional, Menlo Park, Calif., USA) – containing an optic fiber connected to a laser flickering red light source for easy identification of the distal tip through the sclera (fig. 3, 4) – is then inserted and pushed forward within Schlemm's canal for the entire 360° (fig. 5) until it comes out of the other end of the of the canal opening. A 10-0 prolene suture is then tied to the distal tip (fig. 6) and the microcatheter is withdrawn and pulled back through the canal in the opposite direction. A special screw-driven syringe is used to deliver a small and standardized amount of high-molecular-weight viscoelastic agent in Schlemm's canal every 2 or 3 h while the catheter is withdrawn. The suture is then knotted under tension in order to further inwardly distend the trabecular meshwork (fig. 7). The superficial scleral flap is tightly sutured with 6–8 10-0 vicryl sutures to ensure a watertight closure (fig. 8) in order to prevent any bleb formation. The conjunctival flap is then sutured with some 10-0 vicryl stitches to complete the surgery.

The main indications for canaloplasty include primary open-angle glaucoma, pseudoexfoliation glaucoma, pigmentary glaucoma, and juvenile glaucoma.

Contraindications include angle-closure glaucoma, neovascular glaucoma, and previous operations that have interrupted Schlemm's canal,

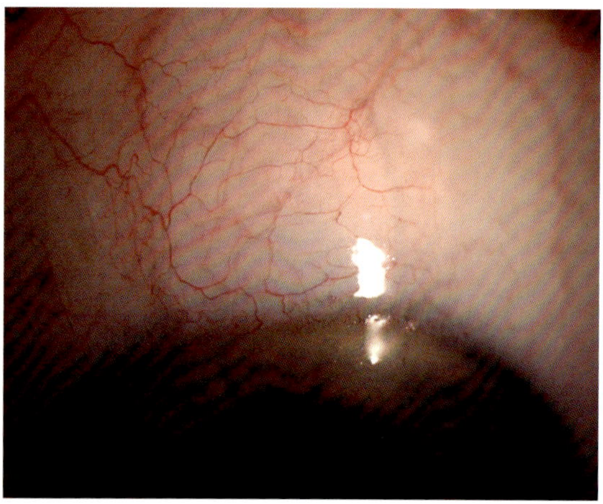

Fig. 9. Eye: 3 weeks after canaloplasty.

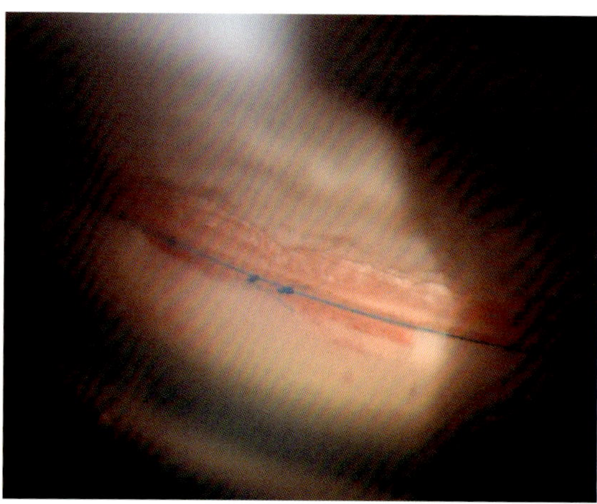

Fig. 10. Prolene suture within Schlemm's canal (gonioscopic view).

even if, in some selected cases, canaloplasty can be attempted with good results [12].

Early postoperative complications (within 4 weeks from surgery) include hyphema, hypotonus, and rise in intraocular pressure (IOP). Patients normally report a transient decrease in visual acuity within the first weeks after canaloplasty, which is due to an induced according to the rule astigmatism that tends to disappear within 1 month.

The success rate is highly variable according to the definition of success (<21, <18, <16 mm Hg, with or without medical therapy), ranging between 36 and 95% after 3 years. The vast majority of patients show mid-term results that are very encouraging, without any signs of serious permanent complications. One of the most advantageous characteristics of canaloplasty is that this procedure provides a reduction in IOP without the need of a filtering bleb, which is currently one of the most critical aspects regarding trabeculectomy. Unlike other surgical techniques, the vast majority of postoperative canaloplasty patients tend to have a perfectly normal looking eye after a few weeks, without any ocular discomfort (fig. 9). The suture can be clearly visualized by gonioscopy (fig. 10), ultrasound biomicroscopy, or anterior segment optical coherence tomography (OCT) even years after operation (fig. 11).

This new surgical technique is also advantageous because of the very low percentage of postoperative treatments needed in comparison to the high frequency of bleb manipulations (up to 78.2% of cases) required after trabeculectomy [13]. Consequently, patients normally require less follow-up visits, which translates to an overall reduction in social health costs [14]. It is worthwhile to note that very few patients (4–7%) have shown not to benefit from canaloplasty, which is probably due to a nonreversible collapse of collector channels that could not be opened based on anatomical factors. Narrow angle eyes, and post-traumatic and other forms of secondary glaucomas are contraindications for this procedure. In these cases, a filtering procedure is by far the best solution. The effect of canaloplasty on IOP, as previously reported by other authors [6], appears to be correlated to the suture tension, and even a modest suture tension (grade ≥0.5) is sufficient to provide sufficient trabecular meshwork distension.

The disadvantages of this procedure include a long learning curve and the need of specifically designed (and expensive) instrumentation.

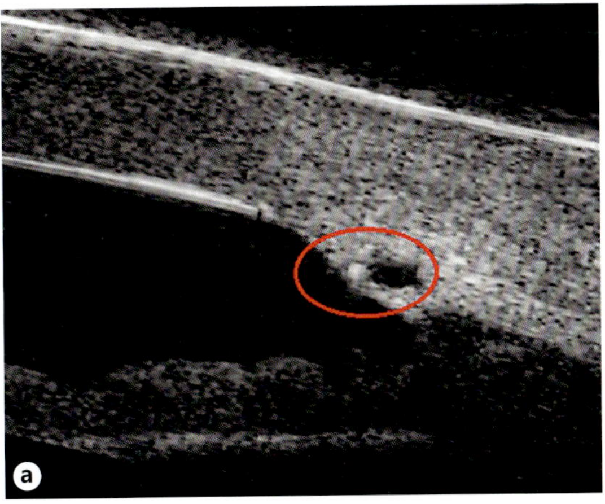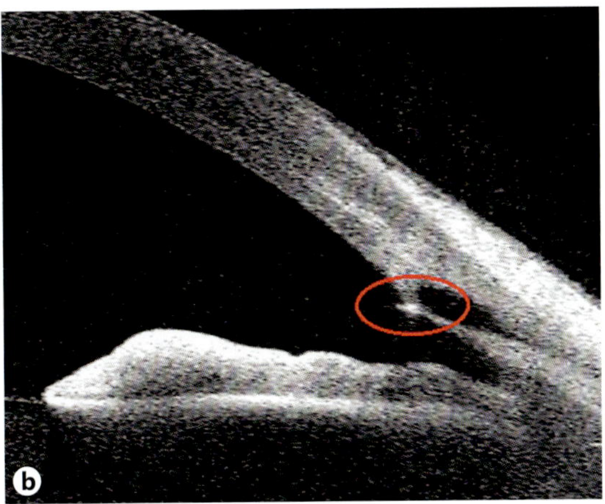

Fig. 11. Prolene suture (red circles) in an 80-MHz ultrasound biomicroscopy (**a**) and OCT image (**b**).

Another limit, especially during the learning curve, is that the successful cannulation of Schlemm's canal can fail at times (about 5–10% of cases), usually due to anatomical factors. In these cases, usually, the procedure can be easily converted into either a deep sclerectomy or a viscocanalostomy, which tend to show good postoperative results. When the microcatheter encounters a stop during the cannulation, the surgeon may be tempted to inject viscoelastic material to open Schlemm's canal; however, this maneuver can cause a rupture of the canal with a Descemet's detachment, especially when the injection is made in the lower sectors distant from the Schlemm's canal opened ostia. This can lead to an intracorneal hematoma when the Descemet's detachment begins to fill with blood arising from the collector channels and Schlemm's canal [15, 16]. Other possible complications include false routes during cannulation, and the passage of the suture in the anterior chamber during the operation or in the early postoperative period, which is rare and usually well tolerated. Bleeding from Schlemm's canal in the anterior chamber can also occur, which can be due to a reverse flow from aqueous veins with blood reflux into the anterior cham-

ber, and thus can be considered as a positive prognostic factor. A rise in IOP can sometimes be found in the early postoperative period. This is due to the fact that Schlemm's canal is filled with hyaluronic acid, thus humor aqueous cannot drain through the trabeculodescemetic window for some days. A YAG laser goniopuncture should be considered before adding medical treatment if the IOP remains high after 4 weeks. Severe postoperative hypotonus is very seldom observed and can be due to an imperfect closure of the scleral flap. This can produce a filtering bleb that should be considered as a real complication, considering that it can prevent the humor aqueous to flow through the physiological pathways, which can lead to surgical failure. In cases of long-term failure, a YAG laser goniopuncture can be performed. If this procedure fails to lower the IOP and medical therapy is not sufficient or poorly tolerated, trabeculectomy can be considered as a possible option, using the previous scleral flap. A recent study compared canaloplasty with trabeculectomy outcomes and reported that both procedures provided a significant reduction in IOP at 12 months [17].

In closing, canaloplasty is a demanding and rather complicated surgical technique, which provides very promising surgical outcomes. The technique is relatively new and literature in this field is limited, thus improvements and future studies are needed to address the following issues:

1 Specific criteria to determine those patients that can benefit from this surgery.
2 Instruments and tools to assess whether or not collector channels are still functioning (this is currently only possible with intraoperative channelography using a fluorescein trace or, perhaps, new OCT technology.
3 Simplification and standardization of the procedure (i.e. a prepositioned suture at the distal tip of the microcatheter, precise criteria for suture tensioning force, and use of effective biologic glues for scleral flap and conjunctiva, for example).

The rate of success is quite high and complications are seldom serious and sight threatening. The main advantage of this blebless procedure is that physiological aqueous humor outflow is restored, even if this hypothesis still needs to be fully demonstrated with appropriate future studies. With these limits and caveats in mind, canaloplasty appears to be a promising surgical procedure which can prove to be an important step towards a safer and more effective treatment on selected patients with open-angle glaucoma.

References

1 Castelli A: Tecnica di 'fistolizzante profonda' antiglaucomatosa (fistolizzazione sotto lembo sclerocorneale, con iridectomia periferica o totale, con, o senza, iridenclesis a grembiule). Atti Soc Oftalmol Lombarda 1965;1:21–28.
2 Cairns JE: Trabeculectomy. Preliminary report of a new method. Am J Ophthalmol 1968;66:673–679.
3 Fyodorov SN, Ioffe DI, Ronkina TI: Deep sclerectomy: technique and mechanism of a new antiglaucomatous procedure. Glaucoma 1984;6:281–283.
4 Stegmann RC: Visco-canalostomy: a new surgical technique for open angle glaucoma. Ann Inst Barraquer 1995;25:229–232.
5 Ambresin A, Shaarawy T, Mermoud A: Deep sclerectomy with collagen implant in one eye compared with trabeculectomy in the other eye of the same patients. J Glaucoma 2002;11:214–220.
6 Lewis RA, von Wolff K, Tetz M, et al: Canaloplasty: circumferential viscodilation and tensioning of Schlemm canal using a flexible microcatheter for the treatment of open-angle glaucoma in adults: two-year interim clinical study analysis. J Cataract Refract Surg 2009;35:814–824.
7 Grieshaber MC, Pienaar A, Olivier J, Stegmann R: Canaloplasty for open-angle glaucoma: long term outcome. Br J Ophthalmol 2010;94:1478–1482.
8 Lewis RA, von Wolff K, Tetz M, Koerber N, Kearney JR, Shingleton BJ, Samuelson TW: Canaloplasty: three-year results of circumferential viscodilation and tensioning of Schlemm canal using a microcatheter to treat open-angle glaucoma. J Cataract Refrac Surg 2011;37:682–690.
9 Bull H, von Wolff K, Körber N, Tetz M: Three-year canaloplasty outcomes for the treatment of open-angle glaucoma: European study results. Graefes Arch Clin Exp Ophthalmol 2011;249:1537–1545.
10 Brusini P, Caramello G, Benedetti S, Tosoni C: Canaloplasty in open-angle glaucoma. Mid-term results from a multicenter study. J Glaucoma 2016;25:403–407.
11 Brusini P: Canaloplasty in open-angle glaucoma surgery: a four-year follow-up. ScientificWorldJournal 2014;2014:469609.
12 Brusini P, Tosoni C: Canaloplasty after failed trabeculectomy: a possible option. J Glaucoma 2014;23:33–34.
13 King AJ, Rotchford AP, Alwitry A, Moodie J: Frequency of bleb manipulations after trabeculectomy surgery. Br J Ophthalmol 2007;91:873–877.
14 Brüggemann A, Müller M: Trabeculectomy versus canaloplasty – utility and cost-effectiveness analysis (in German). Klin Monbl Augenheilkd 2012;229:1118–1123.
15 Palmiero PM, Aktas Z, Lee O, Tello C, Sbeity Z: Bilateral Descemet membrane detachment after canaloplasty. J Cataract Refract Surg 2010;36:508–511.
16 Gismondi M, Brusini P: Intracorneal hematoma after canaloplasty in glaucoma. Cornea 2011;30:718–719.
17 Ayyala RS, Chaudhry AL, Okogbaa CB, Zurakowski D: Comparison of surgical outcomes between canaloplasty and trabeculectomy at 12 months' follow-up. Ophthalmology 2011;118:2427–2433.

Paolo Brusini, MD
Glaucoma Unit, Città di Udine Health Center
Viale Venezia 410
IT–33100 Udine (Italy)
E-Mail brusini@libero.it

Traverso CE, Stalmans I, Topouzis F, Bagnasco L (eds): Glaucoma.
ESASO Course Series. Basel, Karger, 2016, vol 8, pp 97–101 (DOI: 10.1159/000446139)

Phacoemulsification and Glaucoma

Carlo Alberto Cutolo · Carlo Enrico Traverso

Clinica Oculistica, Di.N.O.G.M.I. University of Genoa, and IRCCS Azienda Ospedaliera Universitaria San Martino IST, Genoa, Italy

Abstract

Cataract and glaucoma are main causes of blindness and visual impairment in Europe and worldwide. Both conditions are associated with the aging process, and their prevalence is expected to further increase with population aging. Moreover, both medical and surgical treatment of glaucoma is associated with an increased risk for cataract development. For these reasons, coexistence of cataract and glaucoma is frequently observed. Modern cataract surgery with intraocular lens implantation is an extremely cost-effective procedure with positive influences on quality of life (QoL) measures and visual functioning. Unfortunately, similar success measured in terms of QoL may not be achieved with the management of glaucoma patients with a functional disability caused by visual field loss. Advanced visual field loss may limit visual improvement after phacoemulsification (PE), and a concurrent glaucoma procedure may delay visual recovery. Recent studies show that PE plays an increasingly important role in the management of both open-angle and angle closure (AC) glaucoma. PE, however, can be technically more challenging in glaucoma patients due to ocular conditions such as the exfoliation syndrome, a previous episode of acute AC attack or a history of past ocular surgeries, miotic therapy, trauma, or uveitic glaucoma. Uncomplicated PE alone may serve to lower the long-term intraocular pressure (IOP) in some circumstances. Several surgical strategies exist: PE alone, PE followed by glaucoma surgery, glaucoma surgery followed by PE, and combined PE and glaucoma surgery at the same time. There is no consensus regarding the optimal sequence of surgery; the decision is influenced by numerous factors, including the type of glaucoma, the degree of glaucomatous loss, target IOP, lens opacity, the number of IOP-lowering drugs, patient compliance, the experience of the surgeon, and impact on QoL.

Phacoemulsification in Primary Open-Angle Glaucoma

In eyes with coexisting cataract and well-controlled open-angle glaucoma, phacoemulsification (PE) results in a small decrease in intraocular pressure (IOP; –13%) and medication requirement (–12%), and seems to be relatively safe, although a limited number of patients manifest worse IOP control after PE requiring additional medical or surgical treatments [1]. As filtering surgery could be required in the future, clear cornea cataract extraction is preferred in order to

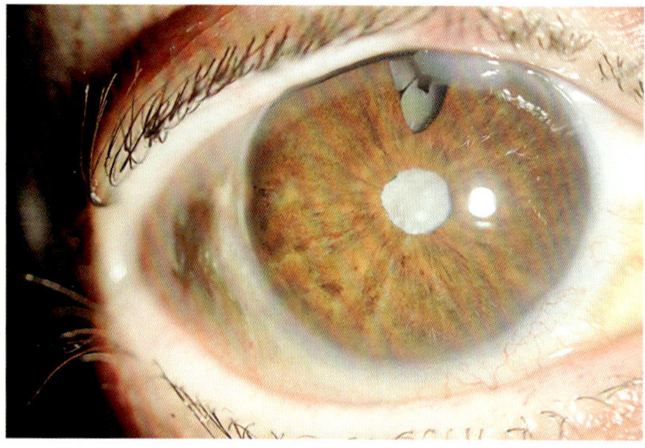

Fig. 1. Dense cataract in an eye with functioning bleb and small pupil.

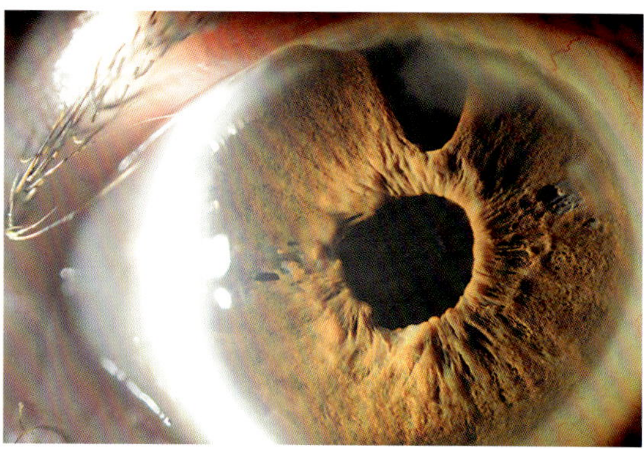

Fig. 2. Postoperative examination at 1 week.

maintain conjunctival integrity [2]. Careful consideration must be given to the severity of the patient's glaucoma because, in patients with advanced glaucoma, transient postoperative IOP spikes may further deteriorate their visual field [3].

Phacoemulsification in Exfoliation Glaucoma

Performing PE in eyes with cataract concomitant with the exfoliative syndrome can be more challenging due to poor pupillary dilation, dense nuclear cataract, and weakened zonular fibers (fig. 1, 2). A careful preoperative slit lamp examination in dilation allows to identify the exfoliation material that accumulates in a characteristic pattern on the anterior lens capsule. The material also accumulates at the pupillary margin, trabecular meshwork, and zonules. Moreover, the trabecular meshwork is heavily pigmented, and the observation of Sampaolesi's line is pathognomonic of the exfoliative syndrome. The pupil dilates poorly and transillumination of the iris may show peripupillary subatrophy. Loose zonules are frequent and predispose to phacodonesis and iridodonesis. A narrow or closed angle is relatively common [4]. These ocular findings are associated with an

increased risk of intraoperative complications such as lens dislocation, capsular rupture, and vitreous loss [5].

Clear cornea incision should be considered, sparing the conjunctiva for subsequent filtering procedures [2]. A pupil that poorly dilates can be enlarged with bimanual pupil stretching, iris hooks, or pupil-enlarging devices [6, 7].

A recent meta-analysis pointed out that in patients with mild-to-moderate exfoliation glaucoma controlled with 1–2 medications, cataract extraction by PE results in a moderate decrease in both IOP (–20%) and the number of drugs required after surgery (–35%) [1]. IOP spikes after PE have been observed more frequently in exfoliative glaucoma than in primary open-angle glaucoma [8].

Phacoemulsification following Trabeculectomy in Patients with Filtering Blebs

It is widely accepted that cataract development is accelerated by any ocular surgery including trabeculectomy, the most frequent type of filtering surgery. Various mechanisms have been hypothesized, such as altered aqueous dynamics, altered nutrient delivery to the lens, inflammation, and long-term corticosteroid therapy, which is often prescribed to modulate wound healing. Also, a shallow or flat anterior chamber is an important risk factor leading to lens opacities after trabeculectomy [9].

PE with small incision and intraocular lens implantation has greatly facilitated cataract extraction in eyes with filtration blebs (see www.karger.com/doi/10.1159/000446139 for online suppl. video). Temporal clear cornea PE is usually preferred because this approach does not alter the conjunctiva and, therefore, minimizes the trauma to the functioning bleb [10]. Iris manipulation may be needed to manage posterior synechiae or a small pupil. Even if in the absence of evidence-based data, ab externo or ab interno bleb revision, as well as intra- or postoperative subconjunctival injection of antimetabolites, are used in selected cases undergoing PE.

In eyes with functioning blebs, IOP control could worsen after cataract extraction, and this risk has been found to increase if the time interval between trabeculectomy and cataract surgery is shorter [11].

Combined Surgery

Trabeculectomy is usually the initial incisional glaucoma surgery undertaken when IOP control is inadequate with medical treatment, laser treatment, or both. In selected cases, trabeculectomy could be combined with cataract extraction, often described as 'phacotrabeculectomy'. The IOP-lowering effect of phacotrabeculectomy seems to be less pronounced than with trabeculectomy but significantly better than with PE alone [1, 12]. Advantages of combined surgery are reduced costs for both the health care system and the patient, faster visual rehabilitation, and decreased risk of postoperative spikes compared to PE alone. Different surgical approaches to phacotrabeculectomy exist. In the one-site procedure, PE is performed through the superior trabeculectomy incision, whereas a temporal clear corneal incision for PE is combined with filtration surgery in the superior quadrant in the two-site approach [13, 14]. In this case, a suture should be placed in the clear corneal incision since low IOP levels postoperatively can compromise the watertightness of the self-sealing PE incision. Intraoperative antimetabolites are frequently used to improve the filtration success rate.

An alternative to phacotrabeculectomy is combining PE with the implantation of the Ex-PRESS™ glaucoma device, always under a scleral flap. This procedure does not require tissue excision or removal, whereas, in trabeculectomy, a corneosclerectomy and generally an iridectomy are mandatory. A quieter anterior chamber was reported on day 1 after Ex-PRESS™ implantation [15, 16].

In patients with cataract and refractory glaucoma with previously failed trabeculectomies, extensive conjunctival scarring or difficult glaucomas, PE could be combined with a long-tube drainage implant. This type of combined surgery does not seem to affect the IOP control compared to treatment with a long-tube drainage implant alone [17].

Phacoemulsification in Primary Angle Closure

Angle closure (AC) is defined by the presence of iridotrabecular contact, either appositional or synechial, potentially leading to elevated IOP and glaucoma. Primary AC glaucoma (PACG) results from crowding of the anterior segment and is, therefore, more common in eyes with smaller than average anterior segment dimensions. Ciliary body size and position, and lens thickness also play important roles. Thus, replacement of the natural lens with a significantly thinner synthetic intraocular lens effectively debulks the anterior segment and has been described to have favorable results in eyes with acute, chronic, and secondary

AC with or without glaucoma. However, since the complications of iridotomy are uncommon, its use as initial procedure is justified in practically every case. Cataract surgery in PACG is generally more challenging and prone to complications than in normal eyes because of a shallow anterior chamber, larger lens, corneal edema, poorly dilated or miotic pupil, extensive posterior synechiae, lower endothelial cell count, and weaker zonules, especially after an acute AC attack [4]. Clear-lens PE for AC has been proposed [18, 19] and a prospective trial is under way [20].

A recent meta-analysis shows that for patients with chronic PACG well controlled by medications, PE alone results in a substantial decrease (–30%) in IOP and medication use after surgery (–58%). Even in the case of chronic PACG with poor-controlled IOP, PE alone results in a marked improvement of IOP control [1]. Thus, lens removal may be considered at all stages of chronic PACG and can lead to relief of pupil block and sufficient IOP control [21].

In a small number of patients, a filtering procedure such as trabeculectomy may be required. PE before or at the same time of trabeculectomy can be considered [22, 23].

For patients with acute AC and clear lens, laser peripheral iridotomy should be performed first but, if the angle does not open, IOP is not controlled, and glaucomatous damage is evident, PE should be considered [4].

Surgical Considerations

Careful slit lamp examination is essential when evaluating cataract extraction in eyes with glaucoma. In the presence of a narrow or closed angle, preoperative infusion of mannitol to reduce the vitreous volume is indicated. Repeated viscoelastic testing intraoperatively may help the conduction of surgery and also minimize endothelial cell loss. In short eyes, iris prolapse is inhibited by placing properly shelved clear cornea incisions a

bit more anteriorly. When peripheral anterior synechiae are noted, PE combined with goniosynechiolysis, which permits to separate the anterior synechiae from the trabecular meshwork, can be used in the hope to free the adhesions and allow for better IOP control. Since glaucoma patients are more prone to IOP spikes, even after uneventful PE, full-dose oral acetazolamide is frequently prescribed for the first 36 h after surgery.

Pupillary dilation in glaucoma patients may be limited by chronic miotic therapy, exfoliation syndrome, and iridolenticular synechiae. Moreover, systemic conditions such as diabetes and α-antagonist systemic therapy contribute to poor dilation. A pupil that dilates poorly, despite the adequate use of topical mydriatics, may be widened intraoperatively using several different techniques. Bimanual pupil stretching using two manipulators can break synechiae and dilate the pupil. Iris hooks or pupil expanders such as the Malyugin ring may be inserted to prevent perioperative miosis. Any manipulation of the iris may increase inflammation, bleeding, and miosis postoperatively. In case of a preexisting bleb, the surgeon should evaluate the status of the bleb because revision could be performed at the time of PE.

References

1 Chen PP, Lin SC, Junk AK, et al: The effect of phacoemulsification on intraocular pressure in glaucoma patients: a report by the American Academy of Ophthalmology. Ophthalmology 2015; 122:1294–1307.
2 Shaarawy TM, Sherwood MB, Hitchings RA, Crowston JG: Glaucoma, ed 2. Philadelphia, Saunders, 2014.
3 Slabaugh MA, Bojikian KD, Moore DB, Chen PP: Risk factors for acute postoperative intraocular pressure elevation after phacoemulsification in glaucoma patients. J Cataract Refract Surg 2014; 40:538–544.
4 European Glaucoma Society: Terminology and Guidelines for Glaucoma, ed 4. Savona, PubliComm, 2014.

5 Sangal N, Chen TC: Cataract surgery in pseudoexfoliation syndrome. Semin Ophthalmol 2014;29:403–408.

6 Akman A, Yilmaz G, Oto S, Akova YA: Comparison of various pupil dilatation methods for phacoemulsification in eyes with a small pupil secondary to pseudo-exfoliation. Ophthalmology 2004;111: 1693–1698.

7 Malyugin B: Small pupil phaco surgery: a new technique. Ann Ophthalmol (Skokie) 2007;39:185–193.

8 Shingleton BJ, Laul A, Nagao K, et al: Effect of phacoemulsification on intra-ocular pressure in eyes with pseudoexfo-liation: single-surgeon series. J Cataract Refract Surg 2008;34:1834–1841.

9 AGIS (Advanced Glaucoma Intervention Study) Investigators: The Advanced Glaucoma Intervention Study: 8. Risk of cataract formation after trabeculectomy. Arch Ophthalmol 2001;119:1771–1779.

10 Klink J, Schmitz B, Lieb WE, et al: Filter-ing bleb function after clear cornea phacoemulsification: a prospective study. Br J Ophthalmol 2005;89:597–601.

11 Husain R, Liang S, Foster PJ, et al: Cata-ract surgery after trabeculectomy: the effect on trabeculectomy function. Arch Ophthalmol 2012;130:165–170.

12 Lochhead J, Casson RJ, Salmon JF: Long term effect on intraocular pressure of phacotrabeculectomy compared to tra-beculectomy. Br J Ophthalmol 2003;87: 850–852.

13 El Sayyad F, Helal M, El-Maghraby A, et al: One-site versus 2-site phacotrabecu-lectomy: a randomized study. J Cataract Refract Surg 1999;25:77–82.

14 Nunn J, Areiter E, Page R, Prum B: Long-term bleb survival after staged trabeculectomy and temporal clear cor-neal phacoemulsification versus com-bined surgery. Invest Ophthalmol Vis Sci 2014;55:6140.

15 Traverso CE, Feo FD, Messas-Kaplan A, et al: Long term effect on IOP of a stain-less steel glaucoma drainage implant (Ex-PRESS) in combined surgery with phacoemulsification. Br J Ophthalmol 2005;89:425–429.

16 Kaplan-Messas A, Traverso CE, Sellem E, et al: The Ex-PRESS™ miniature glau-coma implant in combined surgery with cataract extraction: prospective study. Invest Ophthalmol Vis Sci 2002;43:3348.

17 Hoffman KB, Feldman RM, Budenz DL, et al: Combined cataract extraction and Baerveldt glaucoma drainage implant: indications and outcomes. Ophthalmol-ogy 2002;109:1916–1920.

18 Tarongoy P, Ho CL, Walton DS: Angle-closure glaucoma: the role of the lens in the pathogenesis, prevention, and treat-ment. Surv Ophthalmol 2009;54:211–225.

19 Ho CL, Walton DS, Pasquale LR: Lens extraction for angle-closure glaucoma. Int Ophthalmol Clin 2004;44:213–228.

20 Azuara-Blanco A, Burr JM, Cochran C, et al; Effectiveness in Angle-Closure Glaucoma of Lens Extraction (EAGLE) Study Group: The effectiveness of early lens extraction with intraocular lens implantation for the treatment of pri-mary angle-closure glaucoma (EAGLE): study protocol for a randomized con-trolled trial. Trials 2011;12:133.

21 Trikha S, Perera SA, Husain R, Aung T: The role of lens extraction in the current management of primary angle-closure glaucoma: Curr Opin Ophthalmol 2015; 26:128–134.

22 Lee Y-H, Yun Y-M, Kim SH, et al: Fac-tors that influence intraocular pressure after cataract surgery in primary glau-coma. Can J Ophthalmol 2009;44:705–710.

23 Tsai H-Y, Liu CJ, Cheng C-Y: Combined trabeculectomy and cataract extraction versus trabeculectomy alone in primary angle-closure glaucoma. Br J Ophthal-mol 2009;93:943–948.

Dr. Carlo Alberto Cutolo
Clinica Oculistica, Di.N.O.G.M.I. University of Genoa and
IRCCS Azienda Ospedaliera Universitaria San Martino IST
Viale Benedetto XV 7, IT–16132 Genoa (Italy)
E-Mail cacutolo@gmail.com

Traverso CE, Stalmans I, Topouzis F, Bagnasco L (eds): Glaucoma.
ESASO Course Series. Basel, Karger, 2016, vol 8, pp 102–114 (DOI: 10.1159/000446144)

Antiscarring in Glaucoma Surgery

Ingeborg Stalmans

Department of Ophthalmology, Glaucoma Clinic, University Hospitals Leuven UZ Leuven, Leuven, Belgium

Abstract

Purpose: To provide an overview of the antifibrotic strategies that are currently in use or under evaluation for the enhancement of filtering surgery. **Methods:** A literature research was done and the available evidence was summarized. **Results:** A summary of the available antiscarring agents is provided, going from the well-established antimitotic agents [mitomycin C (MMC) and 5-fluorouracil], over anti-inflammatory agents (steroids and non-steroidal anti-inflammatory agents), growth factor inhibitors (inhibitors of transforming growth factor-β, vascular endothelial growth factor, and placental growth factor) to ρ-kinase inhibitors. **Conclusion:** Although MMC is widely used, its safety and efficacy profile is not entirely satisfactory. Alternative antifibrotic strategies have been studied extensively, which has led to the identification of a number of promising molecules. However, further clinical trials are needed to establish their optimal dosing and potential complementary effects with the existing compounds.

Introduction

Filtering surgery is the most effective treatment to lower intraocular pressure (IOP) in glaucoma patients. Trabeculectomy is the reference procedure. However, this surgical technique is associated with a postoperative wound healing reaction, which leads to scarring and surgical failure in a considerable proportion of cases. Considerable efforts have therefore been made in the past decennia in an attempt to improve the surgical success. Pharmacological enhancement of trabeculectomy using different antiscarring agents was found to significantly improve surgical outcome.

Antimitotics

Mitomycin C (MMC) and 5-fluorouracil (5-FU) have been found to be effective in inhibiting postoperative scarring and are currently known as the gold standards in clinical practice [1].

MMC cross-links DNA and inhibits DNA replication. It can interfere with any phase in the cell cycle and inhibits mitosis as well as synthesis of proteins. MMC has been shown in the early 1980s to significantly improve the success rate of trabeculectomy by fibroblast and endothelial cell proliferation, but at the price of potentially vision-threatening side effects (especially when used at high concentrations), such as corneal toxicity, thin-walled avascular blebs, blebitis, endophthalmitis, and hypotony due to their nonspecific mechanism of action. The efficacy (and side effects) are dependent on the dose, exposure time, and surface area [2–4]. With lower levels of exposure, bleb-related complications are less common, but the incidence of bleb fibrosis increases, which illustrates the trade-off between efficacy and safety.

5-FU interferes in thymidine nucleotide synthesis, resulting in DNA synthesis inhibition and ultimately cell death. In the 1990s, 5-FU was shown to inhibit fibroblast growth. Compared to MMC, 5-FU has a lower risk of serious ocular complications. However, at high levels, it is toxic to all actively replicating tissues, such as corneal epithelium. Comparative studies have consistently shown that MMC is more effective as an antiscarring agent after filtering surgery than 5-FU. Therefore, MMC is nowadays more widely used than 5-FU [5].

Of note, although these antimitotic agents have been used for decades now to enhance filtering surgery, their use for this indication is still off-label in Europe. MMC has only recently been approved for ocular use in the US.

Anti-Inflammatory Agents

Corticosteroids suppress leukocyte concentration and function, as well as vascular permeability, resulting in a diminished fibroblast activity and wound healing reaction. Therefore, steroids are routinely used after filtration surgery.

Theoretically, the use of corticosteroids carries a risk of IOP elevation due to steroid responses. However, although steroid responses are more frequent in glaucoma patients than in the general population, an IOP elevation due to steroid responses is less frequent after filtering surgery, probably because the aqueous humor bypasses the affected trabeculum via the created channel. Non-steroidal anti-inflammatory drugs also suppress the wound healing process but are less potent than steroids.

Inhibition of Growth Factors

It has been demonstrated that a large number of growth factors involved in the wound healing process is upregulated in the aqueous of glaucoma patients, and that this growth factor-loaded aqueous can increase the proliferation of Tenon's fibroblasts by 60% compared to the aqueous from patients without glaucoma. Therefore, these upregulated profibrotic growth factors have been investigated as potential targets for new antiscarring strategies.

Transforming Growth Factor-β Inhibition
Transforming growth factor (TGF)-β is a key cytokine in the wound healing process and has been demonstrated to be present at significantly higher levels in the aqueous of glaucoma patients compared to normal individuals. This growth factor has been shown to stimulate proliferation of human Tenon's fibroblasts and enhance collagen contraction in in vitro models [5].

Extensive research has been performed to investigate the antiscarring potency of TGF-β inhibition. CAT-152 (Cambridge Antibody Technology, Cambridge, UK), a recombinant human monoclonal antibody against TGF-β, was studied by Sir Peng Khaw et al. [5]. In a rabbit model, repeated subconjunctival injections (0.1 mg/ml) on postoperative days 0, 1, 3, and 7 significantly improved the surgical outcome compared to placebo-injected eyes. Histological analysis confirmed that there was less collagen deposition and improved bleb formation without side effects. A multicenter prospective randomized clinical trial was subsequently set up, but, unfortunately, this trial was prematurely discontinued due to lack of efficacy at the used dose (which was identical to the dose used in the rabbit study). It is up to date unclear whether a dosing problem caused the lack of efficacy in the human trial.

Other TGF-β inhibitors have been explored in preclinical studies, but no clinical trials demonstrating a relevant benefit in patients are available until now.

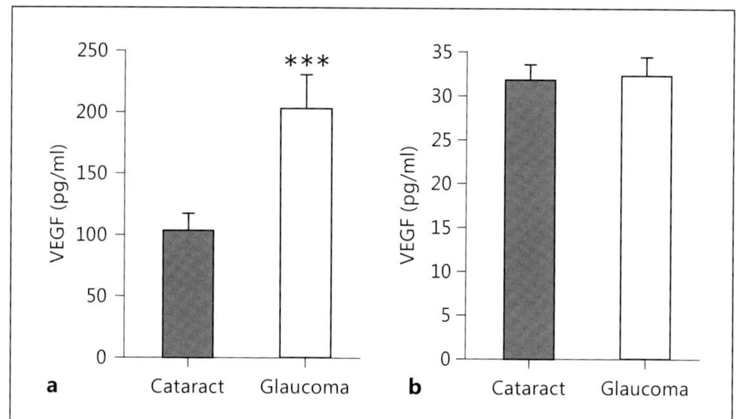

Fig. 1. VEGF expression in aqueous (**a**; n = 20; *** p < 0.001 vs. cataract) and plasma (**b**; n = 10–17; p > 0.05) samples from glaucoma and cataract patients. Reprinted from Li et al. [6, p. 5218] with permission.

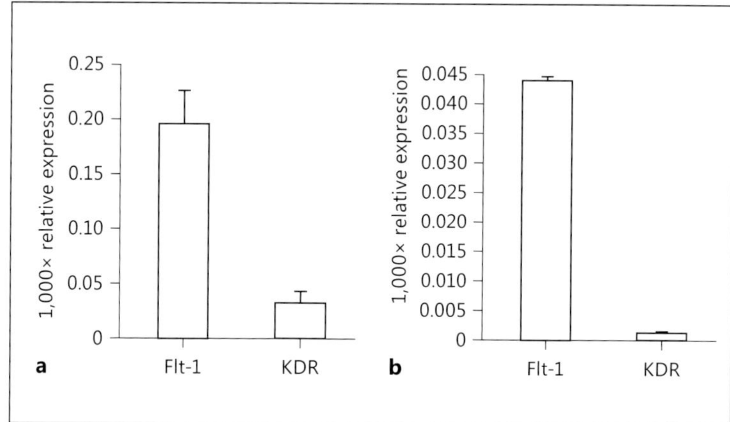

Fig. 2. VEGF receptor expression on human (**a**) and rabbit (**b**) Tenon's fibroblasts. Reprinted from Li et al. [6, p. 5219] with permission.

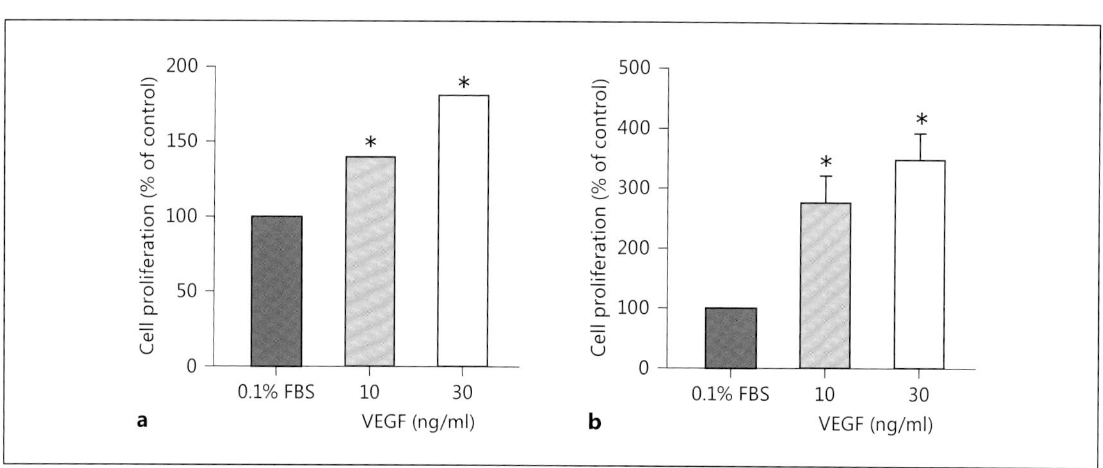

Fig. 3. Dose-dependent stimulation of human (**a**) and rabbit (**b**) Tenon's fibroblast proliferation by recombinant VEGF. * p < 0.05 vs. 0.1% FBS. Reprinted from Li et al. [6, p. 5220] with permission.

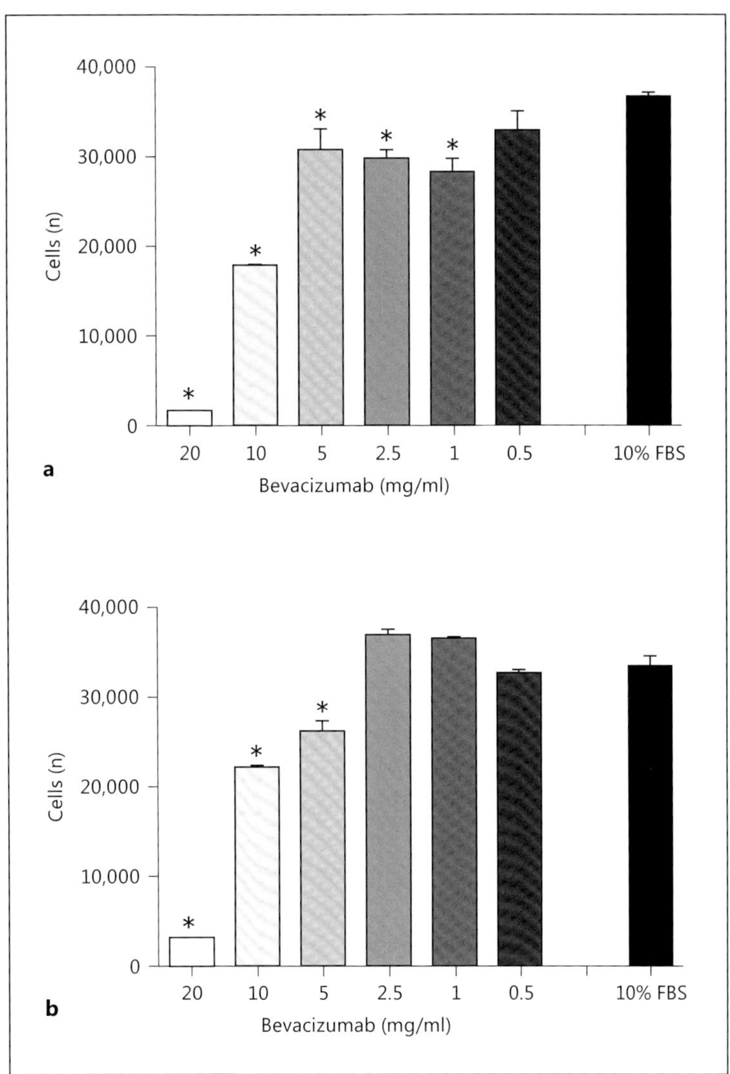

Fig. 4. Dose-dependent inhibition of human (**a**) and rabbit (**b**) Tenon's fibroblast proliferation with bevacizumab. * $p < 0.05$ vs. 10% FBS. Reprinted from Li et al. [6, p. 5220] with permission.

Vascular Endothelial Growth Factor Inhibition

Vascular endothelial growth factor (VEGF) has been shown to be implemented in various processes involved in wound healing, such as inflammation, angiogenesis, and fibrosis. Therefore, the potential of VEGF inhibition to reduce postoperative scarring was investigated [6]. VEGF was shown to be upregulated in the aqueous humor taken from glaucoma patients compared to nonglaucomatous patients undergoing cataract surgery (fig. 1).

Further, cultured rabbit as well as human Tenon's fibroblasts and endothelial cells were shown to express VEGF receptors (fig. 2). In these fibroblast cultures, it was then shown that recombinant VEGF could stimulate proliferation in a dose-dependent manner (fig. 3).

Finally, a dose-dependent inhibition of human and rabbit Tenon's fibroblasts was observed by bevacizumab, a monoclonal humanized anti-VEGF antibody (fig. 4).

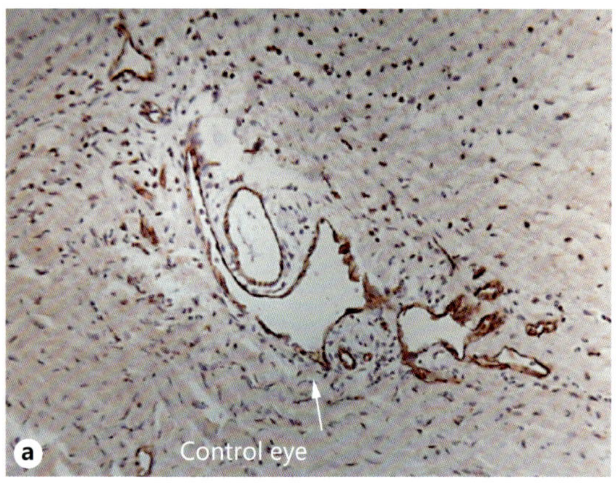

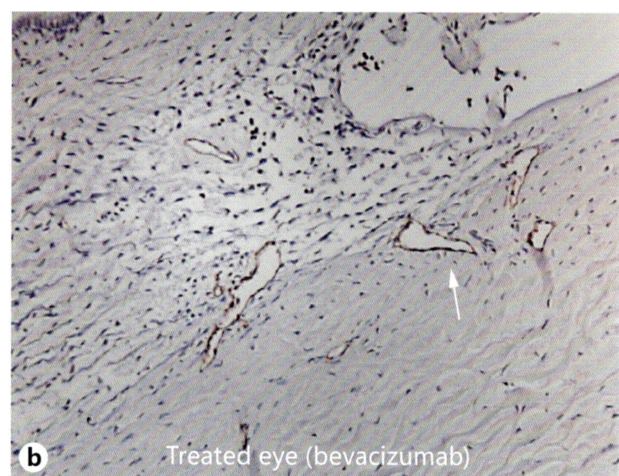

Fig. 5. Reduced number and size of blood vessels in the bevacizumab-treated eye (**b**) compared to the placebo-treated eye (**a**). Reprinted from Li et al. [6, p. 5222] with permission.

In a rabbit model of trabeculectomy in vivo, bevacizumab was shown to increase filtration bleb area. Immunohistological analyses revealed that the blood vessels were fewer in number and less dilated in bevacizumab-treated blebs (fig. 5), and collagen deposition was significantly reduced in the later stages of wound healing (fig. 6).

The effect of pegaptanib (Pfizer Inc, New York, N.Y., USA), a selective VEGF165 inhibitor, on surgical outcome in a rabbit model of glaucoma surgery was less pronounced than that of nonselective VEGF inhibition due to a retained action of VEGF121 and VEGF189. It is indeed known that Tenon's fibroblast proliferation is mainly induced by these isoforms, while VEGF165 has less pronounced effects on Tenon's fibroblasts [7].

Taken together, these in vitro and in vivo studies were strongly suggestive of a beneficial effect of nonselective anti-VEGF as an adjuvant in glaucoma surgery.

Meanwhile, the potential of anti-VEGF as an antiscarring agent in glaucoma surgery was explored in a number of case series and small nonrandomized trials. Despite their methodological limitations, these reports quite consistently indicated that VEGF inhibition could improve the outcome of filtering surgery.

Eventually, a large, prospective, randomized, double-masked, clinical trial was set up to confirm these preliminary results. The aim of this study was to investigate whether a single administration of anti-VEGF could improve the outcome of filtration surgery in glaucoma patients. Patients scheduled for primary trabeculectomy were randomized to receiving either bevacizumab or placebo. Fifty microliters of bevacizumab were administered intracamerally at a concentration of 25 mg/ml at the end of the procedure through a hydrated paracentesis. Patients were followed up after 1 day; 1, 2 and 4 weeks, and 3, 6 and 12 months. The primary outcome was absolute success at 12 months, defined as reaching a pressure between 6 and 18 mm Hg, without the need for additional IOP-lowering medication or interventions. Relative success was defined as reaching the above-mentioned pressure with or without additional medications or interventions. One hundred forty-four patients were included between April 2009 and November 2010 from a single center and operated by either of two experienced glaucoma surgeons, of which 138 patients (evenly assigned to the two medication groups) reached the 12-month follow-up time point (fig. 7). The absolute success rates were signifi-

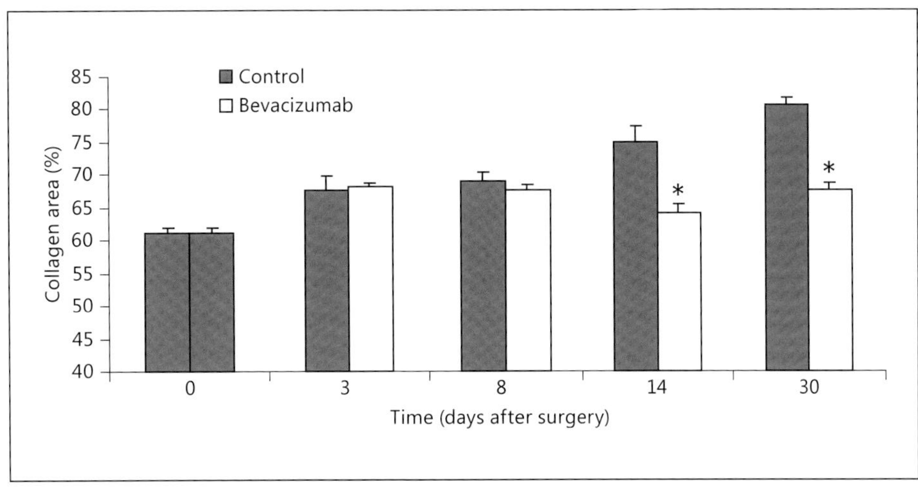

Fig. 6. Reduced collagen deposition in bevacizumab-treated eyes compared to placebo-treated eyes. Reprinted from Van Bergen et al. [9] with permission.

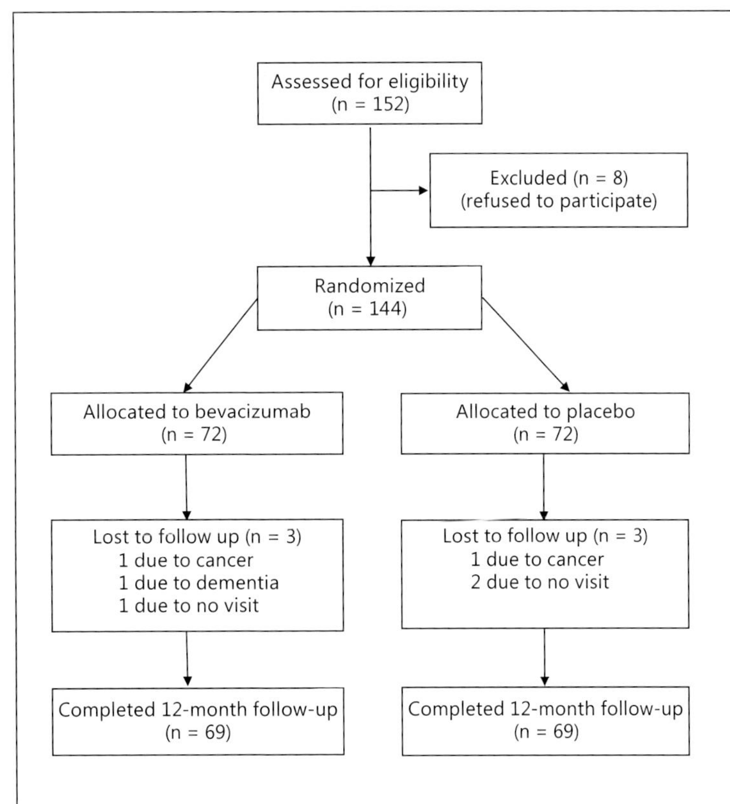

Fig. 7. Clinical trial recruitment. Reprinted from Vanderwalle et al. [10, p. 75] with permission.

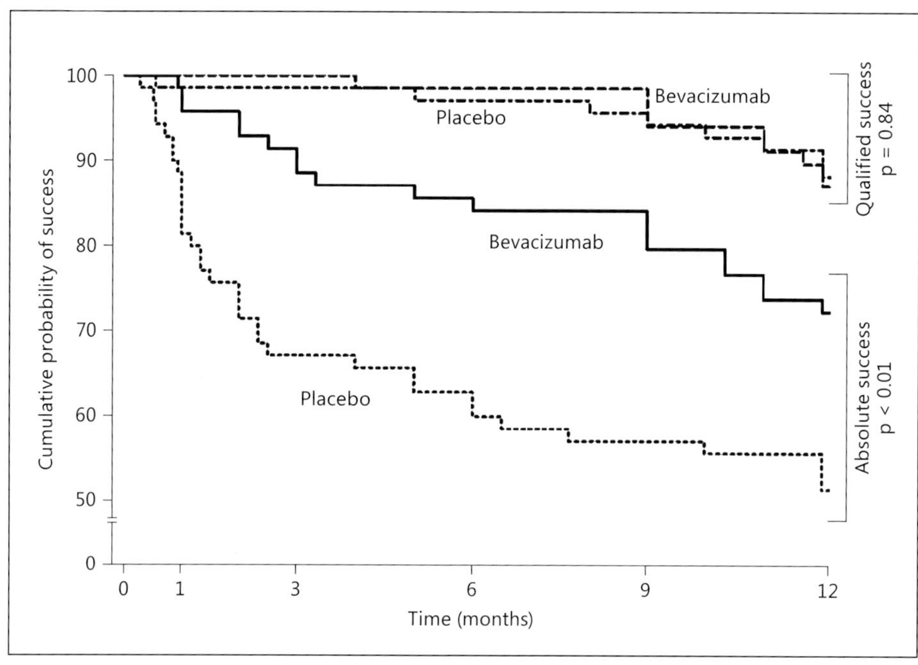

Fig. 8. Cumulative probability of success. Reprinted from Vandewalle et al. [10, p. 75] with permission.

	Bevacizumab (n = 69)	Placebo (n = 69)	p value
Surgical treatment			
Laser suture lysis	29 (42%)	29 (42%)	1.0
Needlings	8 (12%)	23 (33%)	0.003
Bleb revision due to persistent Seidel	2 (3%)	2 (3%)	1.0
Vitrectomy due to malignant glaucoma	1 (1%)	0 (0%)	1.0
Tube implantation	0 (0%)	1 (1%)	1.0
Intracameral tPA injection	0 (0%)	1 (1%)	1.0
Medical treatment			
Patients restarted on IOP-lowering drugs	11 (16%)	15 (22%)	0.51

Fig. 9. Postoperative medical and surgical interventions. tPA = Tissue plasminogen activator. Reprinted from Vandewalle et al. [10, p. 78] with permission.

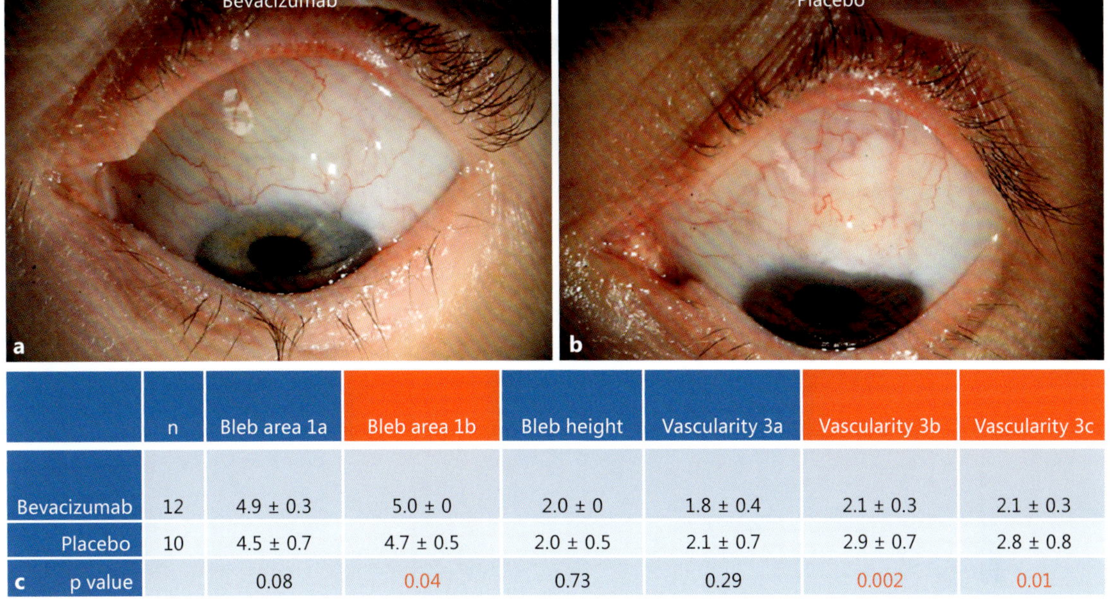

	n	Bleb area 1a	Bleb area 1b	Bleb height	Vascularity 3a	Vascularity 3b	Vascularity 3c
Bevacizumab	12	4.9 ± 0.3	5.0 ± 0	2.0 ± 0	1.8 ± 0.4	2.1 ± 0.3	2.1 ± 0.3
Placebo	10	4.5 ± 0.7	4.7 ± 0.5	2.0 ± 0.5	2.1 ± 0.7	2.9 ± 0.7	2.8 ± 0.8
c p value		0.08	0.04	0.73	0.29	0.002	0.01

Fig. 10. Representative pictures of typical filtration bleb appearance of a bevacizumab- (**a**) and a placebo-treated eye (**b**) at 6 months. **c** Bleb scoring according to Moorfields grading scale.

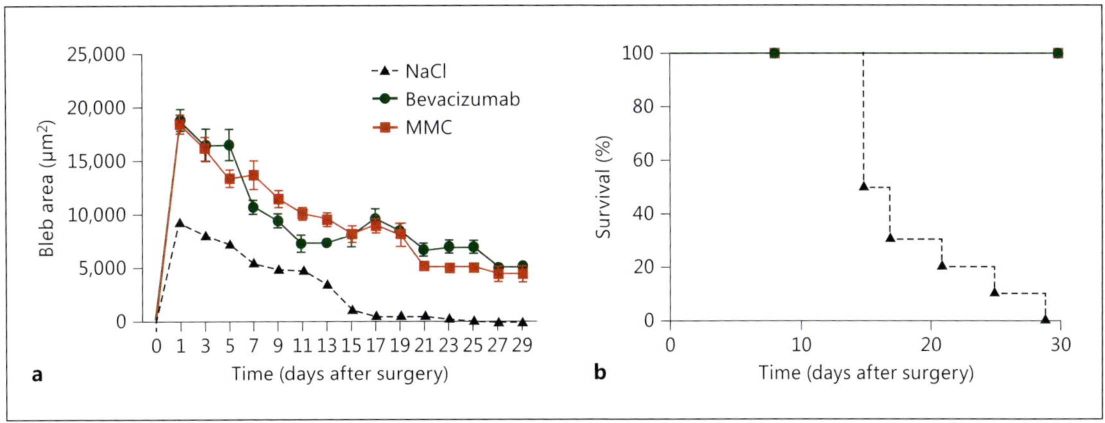

Fig. 11. Comparative effect of bevacizumab, MMC, and placebo on filtration bleb area (**a**; $p < 0.05$) and survival (**b**; $p < 0.001$). n = 20. Reprinted from Van Bergen et al. [8] with permission.

cantly different between the two arms of the study: 71% in the bevacizumab-treated group versus 51% in the placebo-treated group. Survival curves confirmed that the bevacizumab-treated patients had significantly higher cumulative probabilities of absolute success (fig. 8). The number of postoperative needling procedures to rescue the filtration bleb was significantly higher in the placebo-treated group than in the bevacizumab-treated group. The number of postopera-

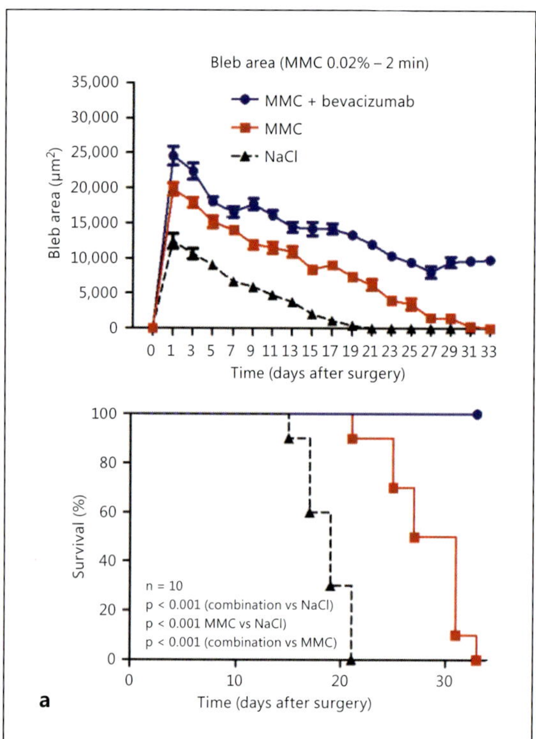
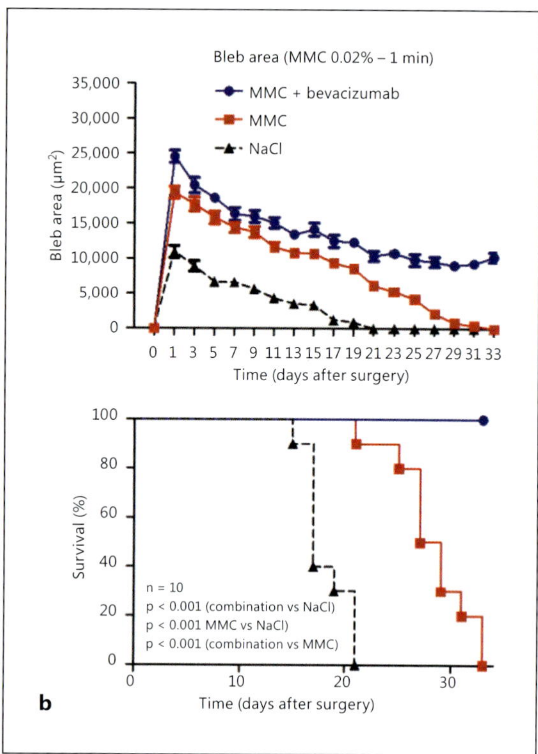
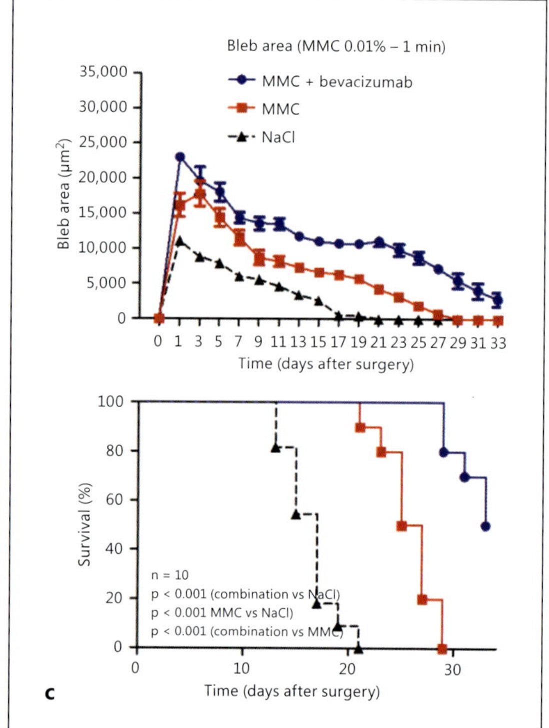

Fig. 12. Complementary effects of bevacizumab and MMC on bleb area and survival at different doses and exposure times. **a** MMC and bevacizumab have a complementary effect. **b** Bevacizumab allows to reduce the exposure time to MMC. **c** Lower dose and exposure time of MMC is less effective. Reprinted from Van Bergen et al. [8] with permission.

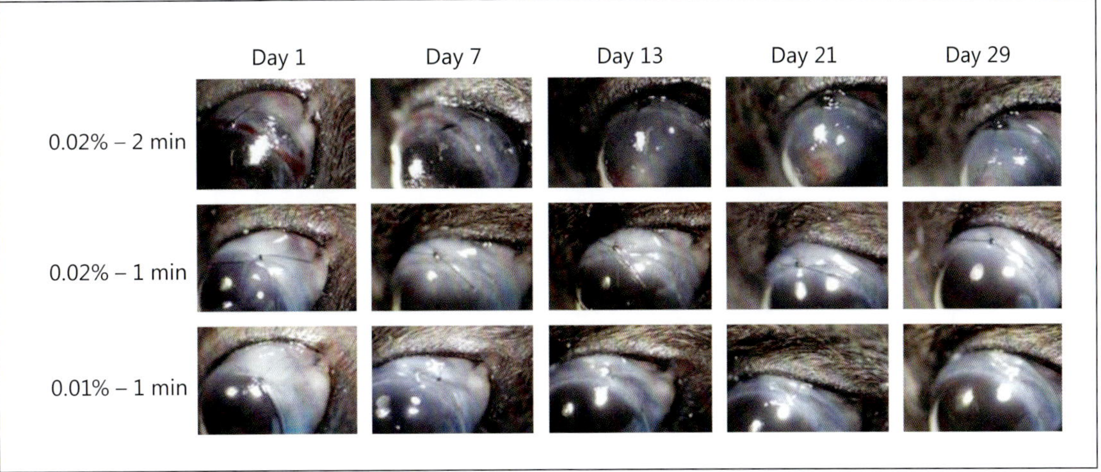

Fig. 13. Toxicity of MMC on rabbit cornea at different doses and exposure times. Reprinted from Van Bergen et al. [8] with permission.

tive IOP medications was not significantly different between the groups (fig. 9).

According to the Moorfields bleb scoring system, bleb photo evaluation revealed that bevacizumab-treated blebs were larger in area and less hypervascular than placebo-treated blebs. As shown on the representative pictures, bevacizumab-treated blebs showed less vascular dilation and tortuosity than placebo-treated eyes, but did not have the avascular and thin-walled aspect observed in MMC-treated blebs (fig. 10). The conclusion of this clinical trial was that a single perioperative intracameral administration of bevacizumab significantly improved the absolute success rates and reduced the need for additional interventions during the 1st year of follow-up after trabeculectomy.

This clinical trial left a number of additional clinically relevant questions open:

1 Is bevacizumab as efficacious as MMC? (Could bevacizumab replace MMC?)
2 Are bevacizumab and MMC complementary? (Do they have an additive effect?)
3 Which is the optimal administration route?

To answer these questions, additional experiments were performed using a mouse model for filtration surgery [8].

1 Bevacizumab was shown to be as effective as MMC to improve bleb area and bleb survival compared to placebo (fig. 11).
2 The combination of bevacizumab and MMC at a dose of 0.02% for 2 min was shown to be more effective to improve bleb area and bleb survival compared to MMC only (fig. 12a). When the exposure time was reduced by half, the efficacy of the combination therapy was maintained (fig. 12b). However, when the concentration of MMC was reduced to 0.01%, the efficacy of the combination therapy was reduced.

Of note, at a concentration of 0.02%, toxic effects of MMC treatment were observed on the mouse corneas. These toxic effects were not present when the MMC exposure time or concentration was reduced to 1 min or 0.01%, respectively (fig. 13).

It was concluded from these experiments that bevacizumab has a complementary effect to MMC and allows to reduce the exposure time of MMC, thus reducing the toxicity of MMC while maintaining its efficacy.

3 To determine the optimal administration route, three groups of mice underwent filtration surgery and received either intracameral, subcon-

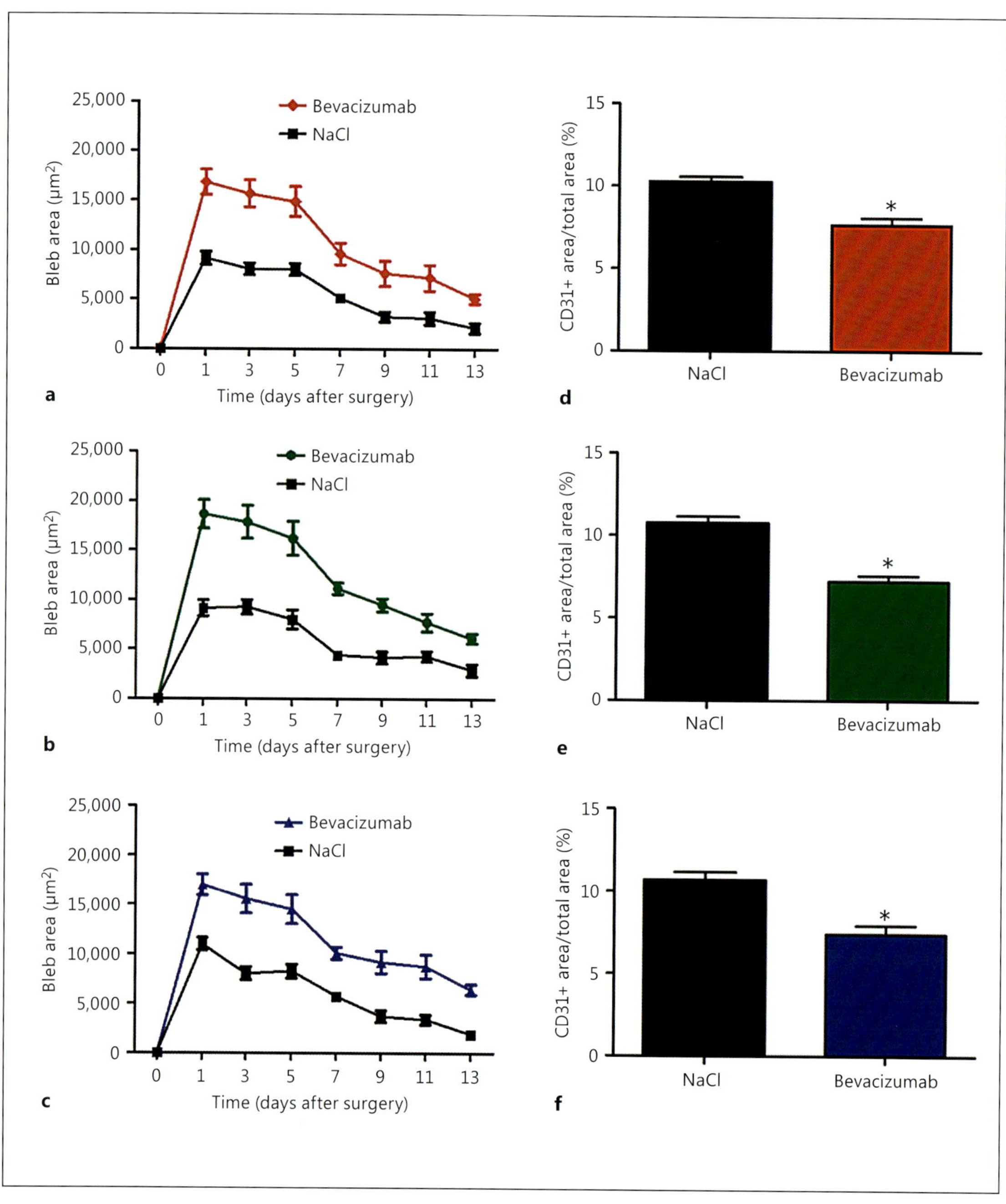

Fig. 14. Efficacy of different routes of administration: bleb area (**a–c**) and blood vessel density (**d–f**). n = 15. **a, d** Intracameral injection. **b, e** Subconjunctival injection. **c, f** Intravitreal injection. p < 0.001 (**b–f**) and p < 0.004 (**a**). Reprinted from Van Bergen et al. [9] with permission.

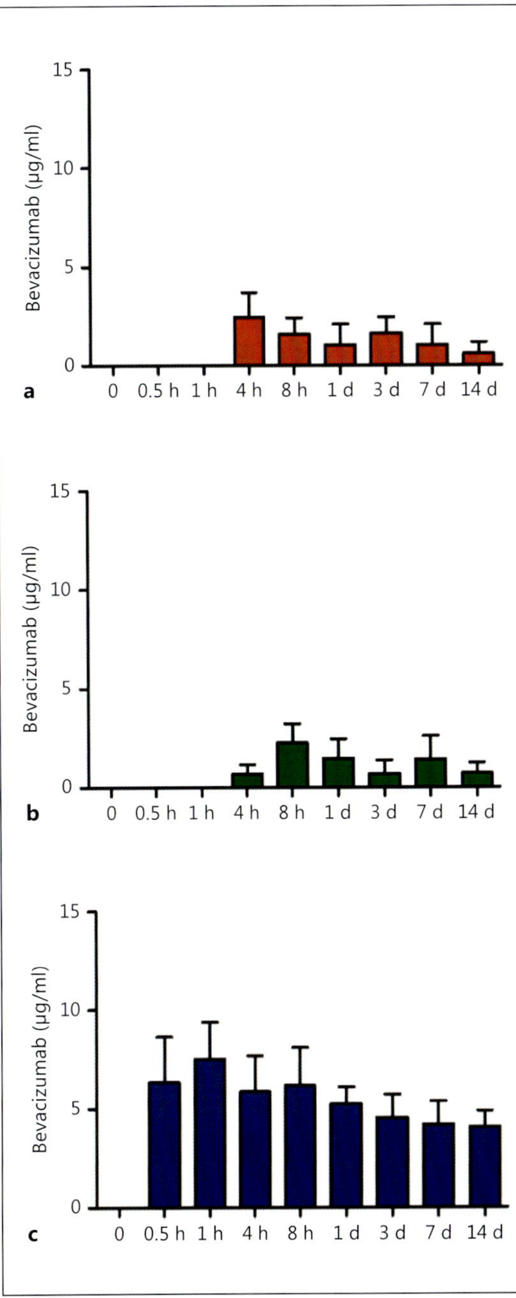

Fig. 15. Safety of different routes of bevacizumab administration: plasma levels after intracameral (**a**), subconjunctival (**b**), and intravitreal (**c**) injection. n = 3. d = Day. Reprinted from Van Bergen et al. [8] with permission.

junctival, or intravitreal bevacizumab. Clinical follow-up showed that all three administration routes improved bleb area to a similar extent as placebo. Histological analysis confirmed that all three administration routes significantly reduced angiogenesis in the filtration blebs (fig. 14). Blood sampling, however, did reveal some differences between the groups. Mice that underwent intracameral or subconjunctival injections showed clinically irrelevant concentrations of bevacizumab in their plasma, whereas intravitreally injected mice exhibited a more rapid and pronounced increase in plasma concentrations of bevacizumab (fig. 15).

From these experiments, it was concluded that the antiscarring efficacy was similar between the different administration routes, but significant systemic absorption was observed after intravitreal injection.

Placental Growth Factor Inhibition

Of note, despite the proinflammatory capacities of VEGF, and although VEGF could improve the outcome of glaucoma surgery by its antiangiogenic and antifibrotic properties, no anti-inflammatory effects were observed after anti-VEGF treatment. Placental growth factor (PlGF; another proinflammatory cytokine) has been shown to be upregulated in the aqueous humor of glaucoma patients, as well as after bevacizumab treatment, which could explain the observed lack of anti-inflammatory effects of anti-VEGF treatment [9].

Intracameral administration of anti-PlGF antibody (Thrombogenics NV, Leuven, Belgium) improved the surgical outcome in a mouse model of filtering surgery compared to irrelevant control antibody. Importantly, the antiscarring effect was more pronounced than observed after anti-VEGF-R2 antibody administration due to its additional anti-inflammatory effects (besides being antiangiogenic and antifibrotic).

Therefore, anti-PlGF treatment might theoretically be more effective than VEGF inhibition [10]. Clinical trials testing this hypothesis are still lacking.

ρ-Kinase Inhibition

ρ-Kinases (ROCK) are downstream effectors of ρ-GTPase proteins and mediate a number of key cellular functions involved in cytoskeleton rearrangement, such as cell morphology, motility, adhesion, contraction, and cytokinesis. ROCK are known to play a pivotal role in various wound healing processes such as inflammation, angiogenesis, and fibrosis. ROCK inhibition has been shown to effectively inhibit scarring after glaucoma surgery in a rabbit model, which indicates that ROCK inhibitors might have a promising place in the antiscarring strategies after glaucoma surgery [11].

Conclusion

Antimitotics have been the gold standard in as antiscarring agents in glaucoma surgery despite their potentially sight-threatening side effects [12]. Growth factor inhibition, e.g. anti-TGF-β, anti-VEGF, and anti-PlGF, as well as ROCK inhibition, might represent promising additions to our armamentarium to improve surgical outcome after filtering surgery [13–15]. Further clinical trials are needed to establish the optimal dosing and potential complementary effects with the existing compounds.

References

1 Van de Velde S, Van Bergen T, Vandewalle E, Moons L, Stalmans I: Modulation of wound healing in glaucoma surgery. Prog Brain Res 2015;221:319–340.
2 Matlach J, Panidou E, Grehn F, Klink T: Large-area versus small-area application of mitomycin C during trabeculectomy. Eur J Ophthalmol 2013;23:670–677.
3 Onol M, Aktaş Z, Hasanreisoğlu B: Enhancement of the success rate in trabeculectomy: large-area mitomycin-C application. Clin Experiment Ophthalmol 2008;36:316–322.
4 Mégevand GS, Salmon JF, Scholtz RP, Murray AD: The effect of reducing the exposure time of mitomycin C in glaucoma filtering surgery. Ophthalmology 1995;102:84–90.
5 Khaw PT, Chang L, Wong TT, Mead A, Daniels JT, Cordeiro MF: Modulation of wound healing after glaucoma surgery. Curr Opin Ophthalmol 2001;12:143–148.
6 Li Z, Van Bergen T, Van de Veire S, Van de Vel I, Moreau H, Dewerchin M, Maudgal PC, Zeyen T, Spileers W, Moons L, Stalmans I: Inhibition of vascular endothelial growth factor reduces scar formation after glaucoma filtration surgery. Invest Ophthalmol Vis Sci 2009;50:5217–5225.
7 Van Bergen T, Vandewalle E, Van de Veire S, Dewerchin M, Stassen JM, Moons L, Stalmans I: The role of different VEGF isoforms in scar formation after glaucoma filtration surgery. Exp Eye Res 2011;93:689–699.
8 Van Bergen T, Vandewalle E, Moons L, Stalmans I: Complementary effects of bevacizumab and MMC in the improvement of surgical outcome after glaucoma filtration surgery. Acta Ophthalmol 2015;93:667–678.
9 Van Bergen T, Jonckx B, Hollanders K, Sijnave D, Van de Velde S, Vandewalle E, Moons L, Stassen JM, Stalmans I: Inhibition of placental growth factor improves surgical outcome of glaucoma surgery. J Cell Mol Med 2013;17:1632–1643.
10 Vandewalle E, Abegão Pinto L, Van Bergen T, Spielberg L, Fieuws S, Moons L, Spileers W, Zeyen T, Stalmans I: Intracameral bevacizumab as an adjunct to trabeculectomy: a 1-year prospective, randomised study. Br J Ophthalmol 2014;98:73–78.
11 European Glaucoma Society: Terminology and Guidelines for Glaucoma, ed 4. Savona, PubliComm, 2014, pp 173–175.
12 Van de Velde S, Van Bergen T, Vandewalle E, Kindt N, Castermans K, Moons L, Stalmans I: Rho kinase inhibitor AMA0526 improves surgical outcome in a rabbit model of glaucoma filtration surgery. Prog Brain Res 2015;220:283–297.
13 Van Bergen T, Van de Velde S, Vandewalle E, Moons L, Stalmans I: Improving patient outcomes following glaucoma surgery: state of the art and future perspectives. Clin Ophthalmol 2014;8:857–867.
14 Lockwood A, Brocchini S, Khaw PT: New developments in the pharmacological modulation of wound healing after glaucoma filtration surgery. Curr Opin Pharmacol 2013;13:65–71.
15 Yu-Wai-Man C, Khaw PT: Developing novel anti-fibrotic therapeutics to modulate post-surgical wound healing in glaucoma: big potential for small molecules. Expert Rev Ophthalmol 2015;10:65–76.

Prof. Dr. Ingeborg Stalmans, MD, PhD
Department of Ophthalmology, Glaucoma Clinic
University Hospitals Leuven UZ Leuven
Herestraat 49, BE–3000 Leuven (Belgium)
E-Mail ingeborg.stalmans@uzleuven.be

Traverso CE, Stalmans I, Topouzis F, Bagnasco L (eds): Glaucoma.
ESASO Course Series. Basel, Karger, 2016, vol 8, pp 115–126 (DOI: 10.1159/000446148)

The Risk of Handicap from Glaucoma

Panayiota Founti[a] · Alexander Spratt[b] · Aachal Kotecha[c] ·
Ananth Viswanathan[c]

[a]Glaucoma Service, Moorfields Eye Hospital, London, UK; [b]Beraja Medical Institute, Miami, Fla., USA; [c]NIHR Biomedical Research Centre for Ophthalmology, UCL Institute of Ophthalmology and Moorfields Eye Hospital NHS Foundation Trust, London, UK

Abstract

The role of health-care providers is not just to diagnose, treat, and monitor disease, but also to promote the well-being of patients. To this end, a comprehensive understanding of how patients feel and function in the presence of a disease or following medical intervention is imperative. The goal of glaucoma treatment, as formulated by the European Glaucoma Society, is to maintain the patient's visual function and related quality of life (QoL) at a sustainable cost. Visual acuity and intraocular pressure measurements, visual field testing, and clinical examination of the optic disc are fundamental to glaucoma clinical practice. Also, new software algorithms to detect and quantify progression of visual field loss, computerised imaging modalities to assess structural damage, and measurement of central corneal thickness have become increasingly important. Despite the value of objective clinical measures, none of these can provide meaningful insight into patients' concerns, their satisfaction with their vision, and their ability to perform visually demanding tasks. However, it is these factors which directly affect QoL and therefore matter most to patients. The purpose of this element of the course is to explain how 'quality of life' has been conceptualised and processed to yield quantitative measures, to discuss QoL instruments commonly used in glaucoma, and to present key research findings.   © 2016 S. Karger AG, Basel

Introduction

In 1948, the World Health Organization defined health as 'a state of complete physical, mental and social well-being and not merely the absence of disease or infirmity' [1].

Although the accuracy of this definition is currently being challenged [2], the holistic concept of health encompassing physical, psychological, and social aspects remains as powerful as ever. The role of health-care providers is not just to diagnose, treat, and monitor disease, but to promote the well-being of patients. To this end, a comprehensive understanding of how patients feel and function in the presence of a disease or following medical intervention is imperative.

The goal of glaucoma treatment, as formulated by the European Glaucoma Society, is to maintain the patient's visual function and related quality of life (QoL) at a sustainable cost [3]. Visual acuity and intraocular pressure measurements, visual field testing, and clinical examination of the optic disc are fundamental to glaucoma clinical practice. Also, new software algorithms to detect and quantify progression of visual field loss, computerised imaging modalities to assess structural damage, and measurement of central corneal thickness have become increasingly important. Despite the value of objective clinical measures, none of these can provide meaningful insight into patients' concerns, their satisfaction with their vision, and their ability to perform visually demanding tasks. However, it is these factors which directly affect QoL and, therefore, matter most to patients.

The purpose of this chapter is to explain how 'quality of life' has been conceptualised and processed to yield quantitative measures, to discuss QoL instruments commonly used in glaucoma, and to present key research findings. This chapter intends to be representative rather than exhaustive in discussing the literature.

Definition

According to the World Health Organization, QoL is defined as 'an individual's perception of their position in life in the context of the culture and value systems in which they live and in relation to their goals, expectations, standards, and concerns. It is a broad-ranging concept affected in a complex way by the person's physical health, psychological state, level of independence, social relationships, and their relationship to salient features of their environment' [4]. The right to drive, the freedom to live independently, and to enjoy life, all contribute to a 'good' QoL, and each of these have a sight-dependent component.

The definition by itself suggests that patients with similar disease states, including those suffering glaucomatous visual loss, are likely to rate its impact on their QoL quite differently. It also implies that QoL may vary within individuals over time based on life experiences and changing personal expectations. However, even with this variable personal resilience, research studies with adequately precise methods and sufficiently large sample sizes do provide useful information about the QoL impact of glaucoma.

With the increasing emphasis on patient-centred care, QoL is currently described under the umbrella term 'patient-reported outcomes' (PROs) [5]. A PRO is a measurement of any aspect of a patient's health status that is reported directly by the patient, free of interpretation by a physician, researcher, or other person. In other medical disciplines, PROs are already being used in clinical trials for evaluating medical drugs and devices. The use of vision-related PROs as key endpoints in ophthalmology, including glaucoma, is still being discussed [5].

Why Is Quality of Life Important?

Being able to empathise with patients by understanding how a disease impacts upon their well-being is essential to quality care [6] and possibly the most apparent benefit of assessing QoL. What may not be so obvious are the implications of this knowledge on a clinical and a public health level:

1 It can provide better understanding of the symptoms of the disease and, therefore, better understanding of the disease itself.
2 It can guide clinicians on history taking and clinical measures that are most relevant to the disease.
3 It can advise on the type of information that should be given to newly and previously diagnosed patients. For example, patients may need to be informed on possible future changes in their lives and modifications to their environment which may help them cope with visual disability.

4 It can guide patient-tailored treatments and promote patient involvement in clinical decision making.
5 It can help identify patients who are entitled to concessions and who might benefit from rehabilitative interventions.
6 It can help determine PROs in clinical trials.
7 It can determine the cost-effectiveness of medical and surgical interventions.
8 It can be used in the development of public health surveillance systems.

Assessment of Quality of Life in Glaucoma

It was not until 1997 that systematic efforts were made to understand how glaucoma affects patients' QoL [7–9]. This young science now incorporates questionnaires, performance-based measures, and utility analyses in its forms of assessment [10, 11].

Questionnaires

Health questionnaires represent the oldest method employed in QoL research. What differentiates them from taking a medical history is that they provide a structured and standardised way to assess patients' perception of their health status. However, not all questionnaires may be appropriate for this purpose. One of the properties that such an instrument must possess is validity, meaning that it has been proven to measure what it is intended to measure. In vision research, this is usually achieved by showing a strong correlation between the information provided by the instrument and objective clinical measures, such as visual acuity and visual field outcomes.

Health questionnaires can be broadly divided into those assessing general health, those which are system specific in their questioning, and those which are disease specific.

Each of these types has been used to assess QoL in patients with glaucoma.

General Health-Related Quality of Life Questionnaires

These were designed to provide a measure of the self-perceived overall health status of a patient and were intended to apply across different types and severities of diseases. Their main strength is that they allow for comparisons of QoL among different diseases. However, because they measure QoL in such broad terms, they may fail to capture certain aspects of QoL affected by a specific disease.

The *Medical Outcomes Study Short-Form Health Survey (SF-36)* was designed for use in a variety of clinical and research settings [12]. It consists of 36 questions assessing physical and mental health status, and their impact on physical, social, and role activities. The SF-36 is one of the most commonly used instruments in medical research.

Studies using the SF-36 in glaucoma patients have found a weak or absent correlation with binocular visual field loss in glaucoma patients [7, 13]. Other studies have had conflicting results on its ability to discriminate between patients with and without glaucoma [13–15].

The *Sickness Impact Profile (SIP)* was originally developed in the 1970s and focuses on functional behaviour rather than on self-perceptions of health [16]. It consists of 136 yes/no statements about behaviours which cover either physical or psychosocial dimensions of functioning. The SIP is a commonly used health status measure across several disciplines of medicine.

A modified version of the SIP has been used in the *Collaborative Initial Glaucoma Treatment Study (CIGTS)*, which is one of the largest randomised controlled clinical trials to have collected longitudinal data on QoL in newly diagnosed glaucoma patients. The CIGTS found no association between reduced functional health status and newly diagnosed glaucoma [15].

Vision-Specific Quality of Life Questionnaires

These were developed to assess ocular symptoms and specific difficulties with vision-dependent tasks. Questions investigating a similar theme are often grouped into 'subscales' to allow for sub-analysis. Examples of such subscales include ocular pain, distance vision, driving, and role limitations, and reflect the origins of these questionnaires in the investigation of the visual impact of cataract. Vision-specific questionnaires are more discerning for ocular disease but do not allow for comparison with differing non-ocular disease states.

The *Activities of Daily Vision Scale (ADVS)* was designed to evaluate self-perceived visual function in cataract patients and consists of 20 questions grouped into 5 subscales: near vision, distance vision, glare disability, and day- and night-time driving [17]. It asks patients to rate the difficulty of each visual task on a five-point scale ranging from 'no difficulty at all' to 'stopped doing because of vision'. Studies have suggested that only the near vision and night driving subscales are statistically independent; the other 3 subscales show intercorrelations. All subscales, however, are significantly associated with clinical measures of visual function [18]. When applied to glaucoma, the ADVS was able to reliably differentiate glaucoma patients from normal controls, and poorer overall ADVS scores were shown to correlate well with the degree of visual field loss [19].

The *VF-14* was also developed to assess functional impairment in patients with cataract [20]. Its questions encompass a broad spectrum of vision-dependent activities, including cooking, reading newsprint, seeing stairs, and night driving. As with the ADVS, it requires the patient to rate the difficulty of each task. When it was originally tested, the VF-14 was only moderately correlated with visual acuity in the better eye, but it was strongly correlated with self-reported overall visual trouble and overall satisfaction with vision.

In glaucoma patients, VF-14 scores correlated with the extent of visual field loss, albeit to a lesser degree than that observed using the ADVS questionnaire [7, 19].

The *Visual Activities Questionnaire (VAQ)* was developed to assess difficulty with everyday visual tasks experienced by elderly patients. It consists of 33 questions assessing visual abilities that are recognised to decline with age. As it has a subscale specifically assessing peripheral vision, it was selected for inclusion in the QoL assessments of the CIGTS, which found overall VAQ scores to correlate with both visual acuity and visual field [15]. The peripheral vision subscale not only correlated highly with the presence of visual field impairment but also showed correlation with the degree of severity of visual field loss in the worse eye.

The *Impact of Vision Impairment (IVI)* questionnaire was developed to measure the restrictive effects of impaired vision on common daily experiences, originally for the purposes of visual rehabilitation assessment [21]. It asks 32 questions, covering a broad range of practical and psychosocial activities. In glaucoma, no correlation was demonstrated between visual field loss and the overall IVI score, although a correlation was found to responses in the mobility subscale. Notably, a quarter of glaucoma patients with relatively minor binocular field loss reported a moderate-to-severe mobility restriction [22] in keeping with previous observations on decreased mobility performance in glaucoma [23].

The *National Eye Institute Visual Function Questionnaire (NEI-VFQ)* was developed to measure the effects of a variety of ocular conditions on daily functioning and QoL. It was originally designed as a 51-point questionnaire and later redeveloped for convenience using 25 of the original questions (NEI-VFQ25) [24]. Both formats have been validated and widely used by researchers to assess ocular disease and, by comparison, to authenticate the results of other questionnaires. When used in the assessment of glaucoma, the severity of visual field loss correlated with the overall NEI-VFQ25 score and the peripheral vision and vision-specific dependency subscales of the original NEI-VFQ [7, 25]. Furthermore, the NEI-VFQ scores of glaucoma patients were lower across most subscales, including driving and vision-specific role difficulties, with poorer scores correlating with more severe visual field defects of the better eye [26].

Glaucoma-Specific Quality of Life Questionnaires

These were developed by incorporating questions specific to the visual disabilities experienced by glaucoma patients. Questions usually focus on straightforward visual ability, specific task performance, and the impact of reduced visual ability on patients. They aim to assess the hidden symptoms which patients often overcome by developing subconscious coping strategies.

The *Glaucoma Symptom Scale (GSS)* is a modified version of a symptom checklist used in the Ocular Hypertension Treatment Study [27]. It asks subjects to score 10 symptoms commonly experienced by glaucoma patients on a 5-point rating scale. Questions are divided into those assessing non-visual symptoms, including stinging and foreign-body sensation, and those assessing visual symptoms, which include difficulty seeing in daylight and blurry vision; it does not assess specific task performance. The GSS is able to effectively discriminate between glaucoma patients and normal controls [27]. Also, the severity of reported visual symptoms correlated well with visual acuity and visual field. However, another study found no association between Esterman visual field scores and those of the GSS [22].

The *Viswanathan Questionnaire*, as named by Iester and Zingirian [28], also consists of 10 questions but asks subjects to make a binary 'yes' or 'no' response [29]. It includes questions about

bumping into things, finding dropped objects, and tripping/difficulty with stairs. This questionnaire evolved from the earlier questionnaire by Mills and Drances [30] designed to assess visual disability in patients with severe glaucoma. Responses correlate well with visual field mean deviation and pattern standard deviation [28] and also with Esterman visual field scores [29], suggesting that this questionnaire effectively targets activities specific to glaucoma. This questionnaire has also demonstrated that even patients with only mild-to-moderate glaucomatous visual field loss have subjectively perceived visual disability [29].

The *Glaucoma QoL (GQL-15)* questionnaire asks 15 rating-scored questions to assess the degree of functional disability caused by glaucoma [31]. The questions used were the 15 most significant predictors of visual field loss derived from an original 62-point questionnaire. These are related to actions demanding functional peripheral vision, dark adaptation and glare, central and near vision, and outdoor mobility. A significant correlation exists between overall GQL-15 scores and a number of psychophysical tests including contrast sensitivity, glare disability, dark adaptation, stereopsis, and Esterman visual field score [32]. The same study also found significantly greater perceived visual disability amongst glaucoma patients with mild visual field loss compared with control subjects, suggesting that early glaucomatous loss is readily discernible to patients. This extends upon the findings of Viswanathan and colleagues and further challenges the belief that glaucoma is an asymptomatic condition in its early stages.

The *Symptom Impact Glaucoma (SIG)* and *Glaucoma Health Perceptions Index (GHPI)* were developed by the CIGTS group with the aim of providing a more complete understanding of the overall impact of glaucoma [15]. The SIG consists of 43 questions, including psychological and systemic inquiries, derived from discussions with patient focus groups and ophthalmologists. Patients are asked whether they have experienced a symptom and, if so, to what degree they feel it was attributable to glaucoma or its treatment. The GHPI involves 6 questions assessing the impact of glaucoma on patients' emotional, physical, social, and cognitive well-being, the stress caused by having glaucoma, and the level of concern about blindness. Correlations with visual field test scores were weak for both questionnaires but showed some improvement when compared with simulated binocular visual field test scores.

In addition to the above, treatment-specific questionnaires have been developed to assess side effects, satisfaction, and adherence with anti-glaucoma medications, such as the *Comparison of Ophthalmic Medication for Tolerability (COMTOL)* questionnaire [33], the *Eye-Drop Satisfaction Questionnaire (EDSQ)* [34] and the *Treatment Impact Patient Satisfaction Scale (TIPSS)* [35]. Although these tools are relevant to QoL, they are described as PROs rather than QoL measures [36], and therefore will not be further discussed.

Questionnaire Scoring Systems: Likert versus Rasch Analysis

Visual function questionnaires have taken their design from assessments commonly used in the fields of education and psychology. In such tests, the scoring system is dichotomous, having either a 'correct' or 'incorrect' answer, with the questions in each subscale becoming progressively more difficult. Calculating the number of correct answers within each subscale reveals the relative aptitude of a student compared to his or her peers. This scoring system is representative of the 'classical test theory' in which the total score is assumed to represent the strength of the trait being measured.

Similarly, visual function questionnaires are usually scored by summating the average score of each subscale to produce a final score of visual ability. However, many consider this approach to be inadequate as visual function questionnaires, unlike questions assessing aptitude, have no correct answer [37]. In addition, many questionnaires use a rating or Likert scale, by which a patient scores the difficulty of each task. These scales represent an ordinal rather than interval scale, with the difference between each score varying subjectively between individuals. Summating such scores does not allow for this difference in patient subjectivity. An additional feature of aptitude tests is that questions testing a similar ability become progressively more difficult, such that higher scores indicate higher ability. In visual function questionnaires, individual questions assess specific visual abilities and cannot be organized in such a way that levels of difficulty are ascribed. Further, averaging patient responses in each subscale may have the effect of masking very different QoL experiences. To use colour vision as an example, 2 patients with equally reduced colour vision may return similar questionnaire scores but if one is a painter this deficiency will have a greater impact on their QoL.

An alternative approach to scoring visual function questionnaires is the use of 'item response theory'. Using this method, responses to questions are mathematically modelled to take into account individuals' responses to other questions within the same questionnaire. This modelling re-scales questionnaire answers in an attempt to remove some of the unhelpful subjectivity of the test. An additional advantage of this method is that test scores are not dependent on specific questionnaires, allowing for intertest comparisons to be made.

The Rasch scoring system is a form of item response theory commonly used in questionnaires assessing QoL in other medical specialties. This system of scoring weighs the relative importance of subscales against each other for an individual. It takes into account an individual's perceived level of difficulty with each task compared with the actual level of difficulty, and so transforms raw ordinal scores into an interval scale. In vision research, Rasch scoring has been applied to the NEI-VFQ and IVI questionnaires, but its use remains rare, perhaps because of its perceived mathematical complexity. With regard to glaucoma-specific questionnaires, the GSS has been Rasch analysed and was not shown to have satisfactory psychometric properties [38]. Conversely, the GQL-15 was recently validated using Rasch analysis in Asian glaucoma patients [39].

Limitations of Using Questionnaires to Measure Quality of Life

Visual function questionnaires have been developed to measure patients' perceptions of their abilities to perform the activities of daily living. They offer an interesting and valid measure of disease severity alongside clinical tests, reflected in the strong correlations between some questionnaire scores and clinical measures of disease severity. They are, however, a highly subjective form of self-evaluation and draw heavily upon patients' own perceptions, expectations, and belief systems. An alternative method of assessing the impact of glaucoma on patients' visual abilities may be the direct observation of how well they perform visually demanding tasks.

Performance-Based Measures

These were only recently introduced in studies assessing QoL in glaucoma. Patients are asked to perform surrogate tasks of everyday activities, such as reading and locating objects, while being evaluated in a standardised manner and with predetermined criteria; for example, these may involve errors, repetitions, and time to complete a task [11]. Performance-based testing offers several advantages over self-reported difficulty with visually demanding tasks. Self-reports are based on patients' understanding of what the presented task might involve, their assessment of the task's relative difficulty, and their own perceptions of their ability to perform that task. Performance-based testing removes this subjectivity and simply involves observing a patient's actual ability to perform a given task.

Performance-based testing is not new to medicine; it is familiar territory in the diagnosis and monitoring of stroke, and other neurological conditions, and is used to assess other problems encountered by the elderly [40]. It has also been used in ophthalmology to assess the effects of the ageing process on visual abilities in the elderly and in studies assessing the functional abilities of low-vision patients. Studies have also looked more directly at the impact of glaucoma on mobility [23] and the ability to drive [41, 42], but none has fully assessed a patient's ability to carry out the activities of daily living.

The *Assessment of Function Related to Vision (AFREV)* is a recent addition to ophthalmological performance-based testing, which aims to evaluate the effect of visual impairment from any cause on patients' functional ability [43]. The AFREV is unique in its use of Rasch analysis to determine a score of functional ability based on an individual patient's ability in each task. Although the test battery is not glaucoma specific, it has been used on glaucoma patients and has shown strong correlations between overall scores and Esterman visual field scores. However, many of the items on the AFREV are functional tests of central vision, and, as this area is often left intact until relatively late in glaucoma, the use of performance-based tests concentrating on central visual abilities may not fully describe the impairments in glaucoma patients with early disease.

The *Assessment of Disability Related to Vision (ADREV)* was developed based on the AFREV, with the aim of representing a wider range of disability, especially with regard to moderate amounts of visual loss [44]. It is glaucoma specific and was validated using Rasch analysis. It involves 9 tasks to simulate daily living activities, such as reading in reduced illumination, recognising facial expression, detecting motion, and locating objects. The ADREV was found to strongly correlate with binocular visual acuity and binocular contrast sensitivity, suggesting that these may be the aspects of visual function that best predict the ability of a glaucoma patient to perform daily activities [45].

Limitations of Using Performance-Based Testing to Measure Quality of Life

Performance-based measures can provide objective information on patients' ability to function and, therefore, are superior to self-reported measures of difficulty with visually demanding tasks. However, they are carried out in artificial conditions, which may not fully reflect the activities that a person performs in everyday life. In addition, they may be affected by a number of factors, such as concentration, motivation, or desire to please or mislead [11], which cannot be measured.

Utility Measures

A common criticism made of the use of questionnaires to assess QoL is that they provide a measure of an individual's general health status but fall short of describing true QoL.

Utility theory aims to overcome the composite approach of questionnaires, instead using preference-based choices to provide a single, patient-derived, numerical value representative of QoL. In doing so, it reveals patients' perceptions of QoL related to a disease state. It has also been applied to medicine as a method to ascertain the cost-effectiveness of medical interventions.

Utility measures are rated on a scale of 0.0–1.0, with zero representing death and 1.0 representing perfect health. A strength of this design is that it allows for effective comparisons between various health states in a way not permitted by other disease-specific measures of QoL. An example of this is that severe angina and bilateral reduced visual acuity of 6/60 have both been associated with a utility value of 0.50, suggesting that these disparate conditions have a comparable impact on QoL.

Utility values can also be obtained from third parties, often with interesting results. In the case of age-related macular degeneration, it has been demonstrated that the general public, non-ophthalmic clinicians and ophthalmologists all significantly underestimate the QoL impact of this condition when compared with the patients who suffer from the disease [46].

Several methods of assessing utility values exist. The two most commonly used measures are the *Time Trade-Off (TTO)* and the *Standard Gamble (SG)* method.

TTO utility values are determined by asking patients how many years they expect to live and how many of those remaining years of life they would be willing to trade in return for perfect vision. The proportion of their future life expectancy traded is then subtracted from 1.0 to arrive at a final value.

The SG method presents patients with an imaginary treatment that has two possible outcomes: either perfect health (or in the case of utility measures in ophthalmic disease, perfect sight in both eyes) with no side effects for the remainder of their life in cases where the treatment works, or immediate death (gamble 1) or blindness (gamble 2) when the treatment does not work. Patients are then asked what percentage chance of death (or blindness) they would be prepared to risk before refusing the treatment offered. This percentage is then subtracted from 1.0 to obtain the utility value.

The *linear scale thermometer* is a less commonly used method of determining utility values [47]. Patients are presented with two 'thermometers'. The first is labelled 'perfect vision' at the top and 'blind' at the bottom, and patients are asked to rate their current level of vision by placing a mark on this thermometer. The second thermometer is labelled 'perfect health' at the top and 'death' at the bottom. Patients are asked to make two marks on this thermometer – one rating their overall current level of health assuming they had perfect vision and another rating their current health as if they were completely blind. Individuals' rating of vision on the first thermometer on a blind-to-perfect-vision scale can then be transferred onto the second life-or-death thermometer to derive a vision-dependent QoL score.

Utility values have been used to assess glaucoma patients. A study of 191 glaucoma patients and 46 glaucoma suspects found that only 22% of glaucoma and 11% of glaucoma suspect patients were willing to trade any life expectancy for perfect vision, giving modest average TTO utility values of 0.93 and 0.98, respectively [13]. These utility values showed poor correlation with Esterman visual fields. By comparison, 12 blind patients from the same study had an average TTO utility value of 0.67, meaning they were willing to trade a third of their remaining life expectancy for a permanent return to perfect vision. A study of 213 Chinese Singaporean glaucoma patients found that most were not willing to trade life expectancy or risk blindness for a glaucoma-free life; their mean TTO utility value was 0.88 and SG for death and blindness 0.94 and 0.95, respectively [48]. By contrast, a study of 105 Indian glaucoma patients found an average TTO utility value of 0.64 unrelated to the extent of visual field loss [49]. The authors suggest the marked difference in their utility value may reflect the severity of glaucoma in their patients and the differing impact of chronic disease and visual impairment in developing countries [49].

A well-recognised weakness of utility measures is that they are prone to cognitive bias, arising from the fact that individuals are required to imagine themselves in a health state that they have never experienced. When people consider the impact of any single factor on their well-being, they tend to exaggerate its importance, what

cognitive psychology terms the 'focusing illusion'. This explains, in part, the widespread opposition to the recent recommendation of the US Preventive Services Task Force against routine prostate-specific antigen screening for prostate cancer, which was decided on the basis of utility measure outcomes [50].

Quality- and Disability-Adjusted Life Years

Utility values provide a snapshot measure of the QoL associated with a particular disease state. That they can change with disease progression or following successful medical intervention makes them suited to longitudinal use. Both the degree of improved health conferred by an intervention and the duration of that improvement can be considered together using the quality-adjusted life year (QALY). This is calculated by multiplying the utility value gain obtained by an intervention by the years of benefit gained. For example, if a surgical intervention such as cataract extraction results in an improved utility value from 0.5 pre-operatively to 0.8 after surgery and that benefit is felt for the remaining 20 years of a patient's life, this translates into 6.0 QALYs gained (0.3 × 20) from that intervention.

When the number of QALYs gained and the costs associated with the intervention are both known, the cost per QALY can be calculated. Treatments costing less than GBP 20,000–30,000 per QALY have been suggested to be cost-effective [51]. Calculating costs/QALY for various treatments allows objective comparison of the cost-effectiveness of various treatments and permits a relative evaluation of the financial merits of competing interventions.

The disability-adjusted life year (DALY) is another construct by which to understand the impact of disease. Developed by the World Bank, DALYs assist health economists in planning service provision and setting health priorities, and can provide a measure of the usefulness of interventions. DALYs represent the sum of years of life lost (YLL) due to premature death and the number of years lost due to disability (YLD):

DALYs = YLL + YLD

DALYs describe the burden of disease to societies by reflecting the loss of productivity of patients and the time period over which that productivity is lost and are another method of calculating the cost-effectiveness of interventions [52]. One DALY can be considered as a loss of 1 year of healthy life. As with QALYs, the cost-effectiveness of cataract extraction has been calculated in DALYs. This intervention is reported to cost 730–2,400 international dollars (ID) per DALY averted in the developed world and ID 90–370 per DALY averted in developing countries. Costs are calculated in ID, a hypothetical unit of currency that has the same purchasing power as 1 USD had in the United States in the year 2000. The Global Burden of Disease Study 2010 recently calculated DALYs in 1990 and 2010 for 291 conditions, including glaucoma [53]. The investigators reported that glaucoma was one of the diseases with the largest increase in burden, and this was attributed to the increase in older age groups in the world population.

Key Findings of Studies on Quality of Life in Glaucoma

Although research on QoL has a long road ahead of it, there are several examples of key findings suggesting that it has already challenged common misconceptions about glaucoma and has provided a better understanding of the impact of the disease on patients' everyday life.

- Glaucoma diagnosis generates fear of blindness in a large number of patients [54]. This brings into question whether the terms 'preperimetric glaucoma' and 'glaucoma suspect' are appropriate for patients who do not have glaucomatous visual field loss.

- Even in early stages of glaucoma, there is subjective perception of visual disability [29]. This contradicts the common belief that glaucoma is asymptomatic until the very late stages and emphasises the importance of early diagnosis.

- Glaucoma patients do not perceive black areas in their field of view or tunnel vision, as is incorrectly shown in simulations of glaucoma symptoms [55]. Such knowledge is important for doctor-patient communication and public awareness strategies.

- Patients who notice gradual visual deterioration are twice as likely to have bilateral visual field progression compared to those who report stable vision [29]. This knowledge is useful in history taking during follow-up visits.

- Bilateral visual field loss causes difficulty with a broad range of daily tasks, including reading, walking, and driving; it is also associated with an increased risk of falls [56].

- Contrast sensitivity is a strong predictor of the ability of glaucoma patients to perform activities of daily living [45]. This finding suggests that contrast sensitivity may be a useful clinical index in glaucoma clinical practice.

Conclusion

The concept of QoL is multidimensional and, therefore, difficult to measure and interpret. Nevertheless, there is a wide variety of QoL instruments which, in the context of carefully designed studies, can provide meaningful information on the impact of glaucoma on patients' well-being. To date, there is no single method that can capture the full extent of what glaucoma patients feel and how they are able to function. Also, no method is superior to the others, because health questionnaires, performance-based measures, and utility measures were developed to assess different aspects of QoL and, therefore, cannot be compared. It is perhaps their combination, as employed in recent studies, which may provide more comprehensive knowledge. At the same time, weaknesses of existing methods need to be addressed by refining or developing new QoL instruments.

To maintain a patient's QoL, which is the goal of glaucoma treatment, we must first be able to measure it and interpret it. Only in achieving this can we hope to understand our patients, comprehend what it is they want from us and at what personal cost, and begin to calculate the true worth of our treatments to patients and society.

Suggested Reading

World Report on Road Traffic Injury Prevention. Geneva, World Health Organisation, 2004.

Barbur J, Chisholm C, Crabb D, Davies LN, Dunne M, Edgar D, James-Galton M, Petzold A, Phelps N, Plant G, Rauscher F, Underwood G, Viswanathan A: Road Safety Research Report No. 79: Central Scotomata and Driving. London, Department for Transport, 2007.

References

1　Preamble to the Constitution of the World Health Organization as adopted by the International Health Conference, New York, 19–22 June, 1946; signed on 22 July 1946 by the representatives of 61 States (Official Records of the World Health Organization, No 2, p 100) and entered into force on 7 April 1948.

2　What is health? The ability to adapt. Lancet 2009;373:781.

3　European Glaucoma Society: Terminology and Guidelines for Glaucoma, ed 4. Savona, PubliComm, 2014.

4　World Health Organization Quality of Life Group: Study protocol for the World Health Organization project to develop a quality of life assessment instrument (WHOQOL). Qual Life Res 1993;2:153–159.

5　Varma R, Richman EA, Ferris FL 3rd, Bressler NM: Use of patient-reported outcomes in medical product development: a report from the 2009 NEI/FDA Clinical Trial Endpoints Symposium. Invest Ophthalmol Vis Sci 2010;51: 6095–6103.

6　Larson EB, Yao X: Clinical empathy as emotional labor in the patient-physician relationship. JAMA 2005;293:1100–1106.

7　Parrish RK 2nd, Gedde SJ, Scott IU, et al: Visual function and quality of life among patients with glaucoma. Arch Ophthalmol 1997;115:1447–1455.

8　Wandell PE, Lundstrom M, Brorsson B, Aberg H: Quality of life among patients with glaucoma in Sweden. Acta Ophthalmol Scand 1997;75:584–588.

9　Glen FC, Crabb DP, Garway-Heath DF: The direction of research into visual disability and quality of life in glaucoma. BMC Ophthalmol 2011;11:19.

10　Spaeth G, Walt J, Keener J: Evaluation of quality of life for patients with glaucoma. Am J Ophthalmol 2006;141:S3–S14.

11　Warrian KJ, Altangerel U, Spaeth GL: Performance-based measures of visual function. Surv Ophthalmol 2010;55: 146–161.

12　Ware JE Jr, Sherbourne CD: The MOS 36-item short-form health survey (SF-36). I. Conceptual framework and item selection. Med Care 1992;30:473–483.

13　Jampel HD, Schwartz A, Pollack I, et al: Glaucoma patients' assessment of their visual function and quality of life. J Glaucoma 2002;11:154–163.

14　Wilson MR, Coleman AL, Yu F, et al: Functional status and well-being in patients with glaucoma as measured by the Medical Outcomes Study Short Form-36 questionnaire. Ophthalmology 1998; 105:2112–2116.

15　Janz NK, Wren PA, Lichter PR, et al: Quality of life in newly diagnosed glaucoma patients. The Collaborative Initial Glaucoma Treatment Study. Ophthalmology 2001;108:887–897; discussion 898.

16　Bergner M, Bobbitt RA, Carter WB, Gilson BS: The Sickness Impact Profile: development and final revision of a health status measure. Med Care 1981; 19:787–805.

17　Mangione CM, Phillips RS, Seddon JM, et al: Development of the 'activities of daily vision scale': a measure of visual functional status. Med Care 1992;30: 1111–1126.

18　Valbuena M, Bandeen-Roche K, Rubin GS, et al: Self-reported assessment of visual function in a population-based study: the SEE project. Salisbury Eye Evaluation. Invest Ophthalmol Vis Sci 1999;40:280–288.

19　Sherwood MB, Garcia-Siekavizza A, Meltzer MI, et al: Glaucoma's impact on quality of life and its relation to clinical indicators: a pilot study. Ophthalmology 1998;105:561–566.

20　Steinberg EP, Tielsch JM, Schein OD, et al: The VF-14: an index of functional impairment in patients with cataract. Arch Ophthalmol 1994;112:630–638.

21　Keeffe JE, McCarty CA, Hassell JB, Gilbert AG: Description and measurement of handicap caused by vision impairment. Aust NZ J Ophthalmol 1999;27: 184–186.

22　Noe G, Ferraro J, Lamoureux E, et al: Associations between glaucomatous visual field loss and participation in activities of daily living. Clin Experiment Ophthalmol 2003;31:482–486.

23　Turano KA, Rubin GS, Quigley HA: Mobility performance in glaucoma. Invest Ophthalmol Vis Sci 1999;40:2803–2809.

24　Mangione CM, Lee PP, Gutierrez PR, et al; National Eye Institute Visual Function Questionnaire Field Test Investigators: Development of the 25-item National Eye Institute visual function questionnaire. Arch Ophthalmol 2001; 119:1050–1058.

25　Jampel HD, Friedman DS, Quigley H, et al: Correlation of the binocular visual field with patient assessment of vision. Invest Ophthalmol Vis Sci 2002;43: 1059–1067.

26 Gutierrez P, Wilson MR, Johnson C, et al: Influence of glaucomatous visual field loss on health-related quality of life. Arch Ophthalmol 1997;115:777–784.

27 Lee BL, Gutierrez P, Gordon M, et al: The Glaucoma Symptom Scale. A brief index of glaucoma-specific symptoms. Arch Ophthalmol 1998;116:861–866.

28 Iester M, Zingirian M: Quality of life in patients with early, moderate and advanced glaucoma. Eye 2002;16:44–49.

29 Viswanathan AC, McNaught AI, Poinoosawmy D, et al: Severity and stability of glaucoma: patient perception compared with objective measurement. Arch Ophthalmol 1999;117:450–454.

30 Mills RP, Drance SM: Esterman disability rating in severe glaucoma. Ophthalmology 1986;93:371–378.

31 Nelson P, Aspinall P, O'Brien C: Patients' perception of visual impairment in glaucoma: a pilot study. Br J Ophthalmol 1999;83:546–552.

32 Nelson P, Aspinall P, Papasouliotis O, et al: Quality of life in glaucoma and its relationship with visual function. J Glaucoma 2003;12:139–150.

33 Barber BL, Strahlman ER, Laibovitz R, et al: Validation of a questionnaire for comparing the tolerability of ophthalmic medications. Ophthalmology 1997;104:334–342.

34 Nordmann JP, Denis P, Vigneux M, et al: Development of the conceptual framework for the Eye-Drop Satisfaction Questionnaire (EDSQ) in glaucoma using a qualitative study. BMC Health Serv Res 2007;7:124.

35 Kerr NM, Patel HY, Chew SS, et al: Patient satisfaction with topical ocular hypotensives. Clin Experiment Ophthalmol 2013;41:27–35.

36 Che Hamzah J, Burr JM, Ramsay CR, et al: Choosing appropriate patient-reported outcomes instrument for glaucoma research: a systematic review of vision instruments. Qual Life Res 2011;20:1141–1158.

37 Massof RW, Rubin GS: Visual function assessment questionnaires. Surv Ophthalmol 2001;45:531–548.

38 Lamoureux EL, Ferraro JG, Pallant JF, et al: Are standard instruments valid for the assessment of quality of life and symptoms in glaucoma? Optom Vis Sci 2007;84:789–796.

39 Wang B, Aung T, Marella M, et al: Impact of bilateral open and closed-angle glaucoma on glaucoma-specific functioning in Asians. J Glaucoma 2013;22:330–335.

40 Rozzini R, Frisoni GB, Ferrucci L, et al: The effect of chronic diseases on physical function. Comparison between activities of daily living scales and the Physical Performance Test. Age Ageing 1997;26:281–287.

41 McGwin G Jr, Mays A, Joiner W, et al: Is glaucoma associated with motor vehicle collision involvement and driving avoidance? Invest Ophthalmol Vis Sci 2004;45:3934–3039.

42 Adler G, Bauer MJ, Rottunda S, et al: Driving habits and patterns in older men with glaucoma. Soc Work Health Care 2005;40:75–87.

43 Altangerel U, Spaeth GL, Steinmann WC: Assessment of function related to vision (AFREV). Ophthalmic Epidemiol 2006;13:67–80.

44 Lorenzana L, Lankaranian D, Dugar J, et al: A new method of assessing ability to perform activities of daily living: design, methods and baseline data. Ophthalmic Epidemiol 2009;16:107–114.

45 Richman J, Lorenzana LL, Lankaranian D, et al: Importance of visual acuity and contrast sensitivity in patients with glaucoma. Arch Ophthalmol 2010;128:1576–1582.

46 Brown GC, Brown MM, Sharma S: Difference between ophthalmologists' and patients' perceptions of quality of life associated with age-related macular degeneration. Can J Ophthalmol 2000;35:127–133.

47 Jampel HD: Glaucoma patients' assessment of their visual function and quality of life. Trans Am Ophthalmol Soc 2001;99:301–317.

48 Saw SM, Gazzard G, Eong KG, et al: Utility values in Singapore Chinese adults with primary open-angle and primary angle-closure glaucoma. J Glaucoma 2005;14:455–462.

49 Gupta V, Srinivasan G, Mei SS, et al: Utility values among glaucoma patients: an impact on the quality of life. Br J Ophthalmol 2005;89:1241–1244.

50 Hartzband P, Groopman J: There is more to life than death. N Engl J Med 2012;367:987–989.

51 Culyer AJ, McCabe C, Briggs A, et al: Searching for a threshold, not setting one: the role of the National Institute for Health and Clinical Excellence. J Health Serv Res Policy 2007;12:56–58.

52 Barker C, Green A: Opening the debate on DALYs (disability-adjusted life years). Health Policy Plan 1996;11:179–183.

53 Murray CJ, Vos T, Lozano R, et al: Disability-adjusted life years (DALYs) for 291 diseases and injuries in 21 regions, 1990–2010: a systematic analysis for the Global Burden of Disease Study 2010. Lancet 2012;380:2197–2223.

54 Janz NK, Wren PA, Guire KE, et al; Collaborative Initial Glaucoma Treatment Study: Fear of blindness in the Collaborative Initial Glaucoma Treatment Study: patterns and correlates over time. Ophthalmology 2007;114:2213–2220.

55 Crabb DP, Smith ND, Glen FC, et al: How does glaucoma look? Patient perception of visual field loss. Ophthalmology 2013;120:1120–1126.

56 Ramulu P: Glaucoma and disability: which tasks are affected, and at what stage of disease? Curr Opin Ophthalmol 2009;20:92–98.

Ananth Viswanathan, FRCOphth
Glaucoma Service, Moorfields Eye Hospital
32 Eagle Wharf, 138 Grosvenor Road
London SW1V 3JS (UK)
E-Mail a.viswanathan@ucl.ac.uk

Subject Index

Urea, intraocular pressure lowering 62

VAQ, *see* Visual Activities Questionnaire
Vascular endothelial growth factor (VEGF), scarring
    prevention in glaucoma surgery 104–113
VEGF, *see* Vascular endothelial growth factor
VF-14 118
Visual Activities Questionnaire (VAQ) 118

Visual field examination
    artifacts 10
    glaucoma defects
        classification 13, 14, 18, 19
        overview 9, 10
        progression monitoring 17, 19–23, 33-35
        quality of life impact 31
    programs for testing 10–12
    techniques 15, 16